KIDNEY DISEASE DIET FOR SENIORS ON STAGE 3

Empower Your Health: Dietary Strategies for Optimal Kidney Function

Sophia J. Smith

Copyright © 2024 [SOPHIA J. SMITH]

All rights reserved. No part of this material may be reproduced, distributed, or transmitted in any form or by any means, including photocopying, recording, or other electronic or mechanical methods, without the prior written permission of the copyright owner, except in the case of brief quotations embodied in critical reviews and certain other noncommercial uses permitted by copyright law.

INTRODUCTION

Welcome to "Kidney Disease Diet for Seniors on Stage 3," a comprehensive guide designed to support you in navigating the challenges and complexities of living with Stage 3 kidney disease. This book is crafted specifically for seniors, offering practical advice, nutritional insights, and lifestyle tips to help you manage your condition effectively and enhance your quality of life.

Stage 3 kidney disease is a critical phase where proactive management is crucial. At this stage, kidney function is moderately reduced, and it's essential to make dietary and lifestyle changes to slow the progression of the disease. Understanding how your diet impacts kidney health is the first step toward taking control of your condition.

Empowerment Through Knowledge: We believe that knowledge is empowerment. Throughout this book, you will find detailed explanations of kidney function, the impact of various nutrients, and the significance of maintaining a balanced diet. By understanding the "why" behind dietary recommendations, you can make informed choices that support your health.

Practical Tips and Strategies: Beyond dietary advice, this guide offers practical tips for meal planning, grocery shopping, and maintaining an active lifestyle. We understand that managing kidney disease can be overwhelming, and our goal is to simplify this journey for you. From stocking a renal-friendly pantry to incorporating safe exercises, we provide actionable steps to integrate into your daily routine.

Support and Encouragement: Living with kidney disease can feel isolating, but you are not alone. This book emphasizes the importance of seeking support from healthcare professionals, family, friends, and community resources. Encouragement and emotional support play a crucial role in managing chronic conditions, and we offer guidance on building a strong support network.

Your Health, Your Journey: Every individual's experience with kidney disease is unique. This book is designed to be a resource that adapts to your personal needs and preferences. Whether you are newly diagnosed or have been managing the condition for some time, you will find valuable insights and practical advice to enhance your well-being.

By embracing the information and strategies provided in this book, you are taking a proactive step towards better health and a brighter future. We are here to support you on this journey, offering knowledge, encouragement, and practical tools to help you thrive despite the challenges of Stage 3 kidney disease.

TABLE OF CONTENTS

INTRODUCTION..2
   1.1 Understanding Kidney Disease in Seniors...7
   1.2 The Importance of Diet in Managing Stage 3 Kidney Disease..............8

Understanding Stage 3 Kidney Disease...10
   2.1 Symptoms and Diagnosis..10
   2.2 Progression and Potential Complications...12

Nutritional Basics for Kidney Health..14
   3.1 Role of Proteins, Fats, and Carbohydrates..14
   3.2 Understanding Food Labels and Serving Sizes...15

Creating a Kidney-Friendly Diet Plan...16
   4.1 Personalized Nutrition Needs...16
   4.2 How to Balance Your Meals..17
   4.3 Tips for Meal Planning and Preparation...19

Essential Nutrients and Restrictions..21
   5.1 Managing Sodium Intake..21
   5.2 Controlling Phosphorus Levels..22
   5.3 Importance of Potassium Regulation..23

Hydration and Fluid Management...24
   6.1 Understanding Fluid Needs..24
   6.2 Beverages to Avoid and Prefer...25

Grocery Shopping and Pantry Essentials...26
   7.1 Kidney-Friendly Grocery List..26
   7.2 Stocking a Renal-Friendly Pantry..28

Breakfast Recipes...30
   8.2.1 Blueberry Oatmeal..30
   8.2.2 Spinach and Mushroom Egg White Omelette.......................................32
   8.2.3 Low-Phosphorus Pancakes..34

- 8.2.4 Apple Cinnamon Quinoa..36
- 8.2.5 Kidney-Friendly Smoothie...38
- 8.2.6 Banana Nut Muffins..39
- 8.2.7 Scrambled Tofu with Veggies..41
- 8.2.8 Berry Parfait with Greek Yogurt...43
- 8.2.9 Sweet Potato Hash..45
- 8.2.10 Avocado Toast...47
- 8.2.11 Whole Grain Waffles..49
- 8.2.12 Pumpkin Spice Overnight Oats...51
- 8.2.13 Low-Sodium Breakfast Burrito..53
- 8.2.14 Almond Butter and Banana Toast...55
- 8.2.15 Lemon Poppy Seed Muffins...56

Lunch Recipes..58
- 9.2.1 Grilled Chicken Salad...58
- 9.2.2 Quinoa and Black Bean Salad..60
- 9.2.3 Turkey and Avocado Wrap...62
- 9.2.4 Lentil Soup...64
- 9.2.5 Tuna Salad with Olive Oil Dressing...66
- 9.2.6 Chickpea and Vegetable Stir-Fry..68
- 9.2.7 Spinach and Strawberry Salad..70
- 9.2.8 Grilled Veggie Sandwich...72
- 9.2.9 Greek Salad with Tzatziki Dressing...74
- 9.2.10 Baked Sweet Potato with Black Beans..76
- 9.2.11 Zucchini Noodles with Pesto..78
- 9.2.12 Low-Sodium Minestrone Soup...80
- 9.2.13 Egg Salad Lettuce Wraps...82
- 9.2.14 Cauliflower Rice Bowl...84
- 9.2.15 Hummus and Veggie Wrap...86

Dinner Recipes..88
- 10.2.1 Herb-Roasted Chicken..88

10.2.2 Baked Salmon with Dill.. 90

10.2.3 Veggie-Stuffed Bell Peppers... 92

10.2.4 Garlic and Herb Pork Tenderloin... 94

10.2.5 Spaghetti Squash with Marinara.. 96

10.2.6 Grilled Shrimp Skewers... 98

10.2.7 Quinoa-Stuffed Acorn Squash...100

10.2.8 Lemon Herb Tilapia..102

10.2.9 Chicken and Broccoli Stir-Fry..104

10.2.10 Low-Sodium Beef Stew..106

10.2.11 Veggie and Black Bean Enchiladas...108

10.2.12 Baked Cod with Lemon and Capers...110

10.2.13 Roasted Turkey Breast..112

10.2.14 Mushroom and Spinach Risotto...114

10.2.15 Moroccan Chickpea Stew...116

Snack Recipes...117

11.1.1 Carrot and Cucumber Sticks with Hummus..118

11.1.2 Rice Cakes with Almond Butter..120

11.1.3 Greek Yogurt with Fresh Berries...121

11.1.4 Edamame...123

11.1.5 Celery Sticks with Peanut Butter...125

11.1.6 Low-Sodium Popcorn..127

11.1.7 Apple Slices with Cinnamon...129

11.1.8 Cottage Cheese with Pineapple...131

11.1.9 Mixed Nuts and Seeds...132

11.1.10 Homemade Trail Mix..134

11.1.11 Bell Pepper Strips with Guacamole..136

11.1.12 Baked Kale Chips..138

11.1.13 Cherry Tomatoes with Mozzarella..140

11.1.14 Smoothie Popsicles...142

11.1.15 Whole Grain Crackers with Cheese..144

Desserts Recipes.. 145
    11.2.1 Baked Apples with Cinnamon..145
    11.2.2 Lemon Sorbet...147
    11.2.3 Berry Compote with Angel Food Cake................................149
    11.2.4 Low-Sugar Rice Pudding..151
    11.2.5 Pineapple Upside-Down Cake...153
    11.2.6 Poached Pears with Vanilla...155
    11.2.7 Almond Flour Cookies... 157
    11.2.8 Mango Sorbet...159
    11.2.9 Low-Sugar Banana Bread...161
    11.2.10 Chia Seed Pudding..163
    11.2.11 Strawberry Shortcake... 165
    11.2.12 Apricot Bars...168
    11.2.13 Coconut Macaroons... 170
    11.2.14 Chocolate Avocado Mousse...172
    11.2.15 Berry Tart...174

Exercise and Lifestyle Tips...176
    12.1 Importance of Physical Activity...176
    12.2 Safe Exercises for Seniors with Kidney Disease....................... 177

Conclusion... 179
    13.1 Encouragement and Support..179
    13.3 Final Thoughts... 180

1.1 Understanding Kidney Disease in Seniors

Kidney disease is a prevalent condition among seniors, significantly impacting their health and quality of life. As people age, their risk of developing kidney disease increases due to various factors, including the natural aging process, chronic health conditions, and lifestyle factors.

Aging and Kidney Function

As we age, our kidneys undergo structural and functional changes. The number of nephrons, the filtering units in the kidneys, decreases, and the remaining nephrons may become less efficient. This decline in kidney function is a normal part of aging but can be exacerbated by other health issues.

Chronic Conditions and Kidney Disease

Chronic conditions such as diabetes and hypertension are major contributors to kidney disease in seniors. High blood sugar levels in diabetes can damage the blood vessels in the kidneys, leading to reduced function. Similarly, high blood pressure can strain the kidneys, causing damage over time. These conditions are common in older adults, increasing their risk of developing kidney disease.

Understanding kidney disease in seniors is the first step toward effective management. With proper care, lifestyle adjustments, and medical supervision, seniors with kidney disease can maintain a good quality of life and manage their condition successfully.

1.2 The Importance of Diet in Managing Stage 3 Kidney Disease

Diet plays a crucial role in managing Stage 3 kidney disease, especially for seniors. At this stage, the kidneys have moderate damage, functioning at about 30-59% of their normal capacity. Proper nutrition can help slow the progression of kidney disease, manage symptoms, and improve overall health.

Hydration and Fluid Management

Proper hydration is vital for overall health, but fluid management becomes particularly important in Stage 3 kidney disease. While it's essential to stay hydrated, excessive fluid intake can lead to swelling and high blood pressure. A healthcare provider can help determine the appropriate fluid intake based on individual needs.

Benefits of a Kidney-Friendly Diet

Following a kidney-friendly diet offers numerous benefits:

1. **Slows Disease Progression:** Proper nutrition can help slow the progression of kidney disease by reducing the kidneys' workload and preventing further damage.
2. **Controls Symptoms:** Managing nutrient intake can alleviate common symptoms of kidney disease, such as swelling, high blood pressure, and fatigue.
3. **Improves Overall Health:** A balanced diet supports overall well-being, enhances energy levels, and promotes better physical and mental health.
4. **Prevents Complications:** By controlling the intake of specific nutrients, a kidney-friendly diet helps prevent complications such as heart disease, bone disorders, and electrolyte imbalances.

Incorporating Healthy Foods

A kidney-friendly diet includes a variety of foods that support kidney health while providing essential nutrients:

- **Fruits and Vegetables:** Choose low-potassium options such as apples, berries, grapes, cauliflower, and bell peppers.
- **Whole Grains:** Opt for whole grains like quinoa, brown rice, and whole wheat bread, which provide fiber and essential nutrients.
- **Lean Proteins:** Incorporate high-quality protein sources such as fish, poultry, tofu, and egg whites.
- **Healthy Fats:** Incorporate sound fats like olive oil, avocado, and nuts with some restraint.

Avoiding Harmful Foods

Certain foods can be harmful to individuals with Stage 3 kidney disease and should be limited or avoided:

- **Processed Foods:** These are often high in sodium, phosphorus, and unhealthy fats.
- **High-Potassium Foods:** Limit intake of high-potassium foods such as bananas, oranges, potatoes, and tomatoes.
- **Phosphorus-Rich Foods:** Avoid foods high in phosphorus like dairy products, nuts, seeds, and processed meats.
- **Sugary Beverages:** Limit sugary drinks, as they can contribute to poor overall health and weight gain.

Diet is a powerful tool in managing Stage 3 kidney disease. By making informed food choices, monitoring nutrient intake, and working with healthcare providers, seniors can take control of their health and slow the progression of kidney disease. This book provides the guidance and resources needed to create a kidney-friendly diet that supports overall well-being and improves quality of life.

Understanding Stage 3 Kidney Disease

2.1 Symptoms and Diagnosis

Stage 3 kidney disease may present with subtle symptoms that can easily be overlooked. Common symptoms include:

- **Fatigue:** Feeling unusually tired or weak.
- **Swelling:** Noticeable swelling in the ankles, feet, or hands due to fluid retention.
- **Changes in Urination:** Alterations in the frequency, color, or amount of urine.
- **Shortness of Breath:** Difficulty breathing, often due to fluid buildup in the lungs.
- **Muscle Cramps:** Frequent cramps, especially in the legs.
- **Itching and Dry Skin:** Persistent itching or dry skin, which can be due to the buildup of waste products in the blood.
- **Nausea:** Feeling nauseous or experiencing a loss of appetite.

Diagnosis of Stage 3 Kidney Disease

Diagnosing Stage 3 kidney disease involves several key tests and evaluations:

- **Blood Tests:** Measuring levels of creatinine and urea nitrogen to estimate the Glomerular Filtration Rate (GFR). A GFR between 30-59 indicates Stage 3 kidney disease.
- **Urine Tests:** Checking for the presence of protein, blood, or other abnormalities in the urine.
- **Imaging Tests:** Ultrasound or CT scans to assess the size and structure of the kidneys and detect any abnormalities.
- **Blood Pressure Measurement:** Monitoring blood pressure regularly, as high blood pressure is both a cause and a result of kidney disease.

Early diagnosis through these tests is essential for effective management and slowing the progression of kidney disease.

2.2 Progression and Potential Complications

Stage 3 kidney disease indicates moderate kidney damage, where the kidneys function at 30-59% of their normal capacity. The progression of kidney disease can vary significantly among individuals, influenced by factors such as underlying health conditions, lifestyle, and adherence to treatment plans. Without proper management, Stage 3 kidney disease can progress to Stage 4 and 5, leading to severe kidney damage and potentially necessitating dialysis or a kidney transplant.

Factors Contributing to Progression

Several factors can accelerate the progression of kidney disease, including:

- **Poor Blood Pressure Control:** Uncontrolled high blood pressure can cause further damage to the kidneys.
- **Unmanaged Diabetes:** High blood sugar levels can exacerbate kidney damage.
- **High Protein Intake:** Excessive protein consumption can strain the kidneys.
- **Smoking:** Smoking can demolish kidney capability and by and large wellbeing.
- **Inadequate Hydration:** Dehydration can impair kidney function and contribute to damage.

Potential Complications

As kidney disease progresses, several complications can arise, impacting overall health and quality of life:

1. **Cardiovascular Disease:** Kidney disease increases the risk of heart disease, including heart attacks and strokes, due to the interplay between the kidneys and the cardiovascular system.
2. **Anemia:** Reduced kidney function can lead to anemia, causing fatigue, weakness, and other related symptoms.
3. **Bone Disease:** Imbalances in calcium and phosphorus can result in weakened bones, increasing the risk of fractures and osteoporosis.

4. **Electrolyte Imbalances:** The kidneys regulate electrolytes like potassium and sodium. Impaired function can lead to dangerous imbalances, affecting heart and muscle function.
5. **Fluid Retention:** Poor kidney function can cause fluid buildup, leading to swelling, high blood pressure, and shortness of breath.
6. **Metabolic Acidosis:** The kidneys assist with keeping up with the body's corrosive base equilibrium. Brokenness can prompt acidosis, causing weakness, turmoil, and muscle breakdown.
7. **Uremia:** Severe buildup of waste products in the blood can lead to uremia, causing nausea, vomiting, difficulty concentrating, and severe itching.

Preventing Complications

Preventing complications involves proactive management and lifestyle modifications:

- **Adhering to a Kidney-Friendly Diet:** Following dietary guidelines to reduce strain on the kidneys and manage nutrient intake.
- **Monitoring Blood Pressure and Blood Sugar:** Regularly checking and managing blood pressure and blood sugar levels to prevent further damage.
- **Staying Hydrated:** Drinking adequate fluids, as advised by healthcare providers, to support kidney function.
- **Regular Medical Check-Ups:** Frequent visits to healthcare providers for monitoring and early detection of potential complications.
- **Medication Management:** Taking prescribed medications correctly to manage blood pressure, diabetes, and other related conditions.

Understanding the progression and potential complications of Stage 3 kidney disease is crucial for effective management. By adopting a proactive approach, including dietary changes, lifestyle modifications, and regular medical care, individuals can slow disease progression and reduce the risk of complications, thereby enhancing their overall health and quality of life.

Nutritional Basics for Kidney Health

3.1 Role of Proteins, Fats, and Carbohydrates

Proteins: Proteins are essential for building and repairing tissues, maintaining muscle mass, and supporting immune function. However, in Stage 3 kidney disease, it's crucial to consume moderate amounts of high-quality protein to avoid putting extra strain on the kidneys. Sources like lean meats, fish, poultry, and plant-based proteins are recommended.

Fats: Fats provide a concentrated source of energy and help absorb fat-soluble vitamins. Healthy fats, such as those found in olive oil, avocados, and nuts, support heart health and reduce inflammation. It's important to limit saturated and trans fats, which can contribute to cardiovascular disease, a common complication of kidney disease.

Carbohydrates: Carbohydrates are the body's primary energy source. Choosing complex carbohydrates, like whole grains, vegetables, and fruits, can provide sustained energy and essential nutrients. It's essential to manage carbohydrate intake, especially for those with diabetes, to maintain stable blood sugar levels and prevent additional kidney stress.

Balancing these macronutrients appropriately can help manage Stage 3 kidney disease and promote overall health.

3.2 Understanding Food Labels and Serving Sizes

Understanding Food Labels: Reading food labels is crucial for managing kidney disease. Look for information on sodium, protein, potassium, and phosphorus content. Pay attention to the serving size listed on the label, as nutrient values are based on this specific amount. Choose products with lower sodium and phosphorus levels to reduce strain on the kidneys.

Serving Sizes: Serving sizes help control nutrient intake and maintain a balanced diet. Measure portions accurately to ensure you're not consuming more than recommended, especially for protein and high-potassium foods. Familiarize yourself with standard serving sizes for various food groups to make better dietary choices and manage kidney health effectively.

Creating a Kidney-Friendly Diet Plan

4.1 Personalized Nutrition Needs

Personalized nutrition is essential for managing Stage 3 kidney disease effectively. Each individual's dietary needs can vary based on factors such as age, weight, activity level, and other underlying health conditions. Consulting with a registered dietitian or healthcare provider can help tailor a nutrition plan that meets your specific requirements, ensuring adequate nutrient intake while minimizing kidney stress. This personalized approach helps in maintaining overall health, managing symptoms, and slowing the progression of kidney disease.

4.2 How to Balance Your Meals

Balancing your meals is key to managing Stage 3 kidney disease effectively. A well-balanced meal provides the necessary nutrients without overburdening your kidneys. Here are some guidelines to help you create balanced meals:

1. Portion Control: Understanding portion sizes helps regulate nutrient intake. Use measuring cups, spoons, and food scales to ensure you're eating appropriate amounts of each food group.

2. Plate Method: Visualize your plate divided into sections to balance your meal:

- Half of your plate with non-starchy vegetables (e.g., bell peppers, cauliflower, lettuce).
- A quarter of your plate with lean protein (e.g., fish, chicken, tofu).
- A quarter of your plate with whole grains or starchy vegetables (e.g., brown rice, quinoa, sweet potatoes).

3. Protein: Choose high-quality protein sources in moderate amounts. Opt for lean meats, poultry, fish, eggs, and plant-based proteins like beans and legumes. Limit high-protein foods that can strain the kidneys.

4. Carbohydrates: Select complex carbohydrates that provide fiber and sustained energy. Whole grains, fruits, and vegetables are excellent choices. Limit simple sugars and refined carbs to maintain stable blood sugar levels.

5. Healthy Fats: Consolidate solid fats from sources like olive oil, avocados, nuts, and seeds. Avoid saturated and trans fats found in processed and fried foods, as they can contribute to heart disease.

6. Sodium: Reduce sodium intake by avoiding processed foods, canned goods, and restaurant meals. Use spices and flavors to enhance your dinners rather than salt. Aim for fresh, whole foods whenever possible.

7. Potassium and Phosphorus: Monitor and manage intake of these minerals. Choose low-potassium fruits and vegetables, and limit high-phosphorus foods such as dairy products, nuts, and certain beverages.

8. Hydration: Maintain proper hydration by drinking adequate fluids, but avoid overconsumption. Follow your healthcare provider's advice on the appropriate amount of fluid intake based on your condition.

9. Meal Planning: Plan your meals in advance to ensure they are balanced and kidney-friendly. Create a weekly menu, make a grocery list, and prepare meals at home to control ingredients and portion sizes.

10. Reading Labels: Learn to read food labels to check for nutrient content, particularly sodium, potassium, and phosphorus. Choose products with lower levels of these nutrients to better manage your kidney health.

By following these guidelines, you can create balanced meals that support your kidney health, manage symptoms, and improve overall well-being. Balancing your meals appropriately helps to slow the progression of Stage 3 kidney disease and enhances your quality of life.

4.3 Tips for Meal Planning and Preparation

Effective meal planning and preparation are crucial for managing Stage 3 kidney disease. By organizing your meals in advance, you can ensure they are balanced, nutritious, and kidney-friendly. Here are some tips to help you plan and prepare meals:

1. Plan Your Meals Weekly: Create a weekly meal plan that includes breakfast, lunch, dinner, and snacks. This helps you stay organized and ensures you have all the ingredients you need. Consider your dietary restrictions and nutrient needs when planning.

2. Make a Shopping List: Based on your meal plan, make a detailed shopping list. Stick to the list while shopping to avoid impulse buys that may not align with your dietary needs. Focus on fresh, whole foods and avoid processed items high in sodium, potassium, and phosphorus.

3. Batch Cooking: Prepare larger quantities of meals and divide them into individual portions. Store these portions in the refrigerator or freezer for quick, easy access throughout the week. Batch cooking saves time and ensures you always have a healthy meal ready.

4. Use Kidney-Friendly Recipes: Find recipes that cater to your dietary needs. Look for cookbooks or online resources specifically designed for people with kidney disease. These recipes typically include nutrient information and portion sizes that align with your restrictions.

5. Pre-Prepare Ingredients: Chop vegetables, marinate proteins, and measure out portions in advance. Having pre-prepared ingredients makes cooking quicker and less stressful, especially on busy days.

6. Focus on Variety: Include a variety of foods in your meal plan to ensure you get a wide range of nutrients. Rotate different proteins, grains, fruits, and vegetables to keep meals interesting and nutritionally balanced.

7. Control Portions: Use measuring cups, spoons, and a kitchen scale to control portion sizes. This is especially important for high-protein foods, high-potassium vegetables, and high-phosphorus items. Consistent portion control helps manage nutrient intake effectively.

8. Healthy Snacks: Plan for kidney-friendly snacks such as apple slices with almond butter, cucumber sticks, or low-sodium popcorn. Having healthy snacks on hand prevents reaching for unhealthy options when hunger strikes.

9. Stay Hydrated: Include fluids in your meal plan. While fluid needs vary for each person, it's essential to drink enough to stay hydrated without overloading your kidneys. Discuss your fluid intake with your healthcare provider.

10. Adjust Recipes: Modify favorite recipes to fit your dietary needs. Reduce sodium by using herbs and spices for flavor. Choose lower-potassium vegetables and adjust portion sizes of protein and high-phosphorus foods.

11. Use Tools and Resources: Utilize meal planning apps or websites that offer kidney-friendly meal plans and recipes. These tools can simplify the planning process and provide new ideas for balanced meals.

12. Involve Family: If you live with family, involve them in meal planning and preparation. This ensures everyone understands and supports your dietary needs. Cooking together can also be a fun and collaborative activity.

By following these tips for meal planning and preparation, you can create meals that support your kidney health, manage symptoms, and provide balanced nutrition. Planning ahead and being organized in the kitchen can make a significant difference in managing Stage 3 kidney disease effectively.

Essential Nutrients and Restrictions

5.1 Managing Sodium Intake

Managing sodium intake is essential for individuals with Stage 3 kidney disease. Excessive sodium can lead to high blood pressure and fluid retention, worsening kidney function. Here are some tips for managing sodium intake:

- **Choose Fresh Foods:** Opt for fresh fruits, vegetables, and unprocessed meats, which are naturally low in sodium.
- **Read Food Labels:** Check labels for sodium content and select low-sodium or no-salt-added options.
- **Cook at Home:** Prepare meals at home to control the amount of salt used. Use spices and flavors for flavor rather than salt.
- **Avoid Processed Foods:** Limit intake of canned soups, frozen meals, snack foods, and deli meats, which are often high in sodium.
- **Rinse Canned Foods:** If you use canned vegetables or beans, rinse them under water to reduce sodium content.

By making these adjustments, you can better manage your sodium intake and support kidney health.

5.2 Controlling Phosphorus Levels

Controlling phosphorus levels is crucial for managing Stage 3 kidney disease, as high phosphorus can lead to bone and heart problems. Here are some tips:

- **Limit High-Phosphorus Foods:** Reduce intake of dairy products, nuts, seeds, beans, and organ meats.
- **Choose Low-Phosphorus Alternatives:** Opt for non-dairy milk (such as almond or rice milk), fresh fruits, and vegetables.
- **Check Food Labels:** Avoid foods with added phosphates, often listed as "phosphate" or "phosphoric acid" on labels.
- **Take Phosphate Binders:** If prescribed by your doctor, take phosphate binders with meals to help control phosphorus absorption.

By monitoring and managing phosphorus intake, you can help protect your bones and cardiovascular health.

5.3 Importance of Potassium Regulation

Regulating potassium levels is vital for individuals with Stage 3 kidney disease, as the kidneys' ability to balance potassium diminishes. High potassium can lead to serious heart problems. Here are some tips:

- **Monitor Potassium Intake:** Be mindful of high-potassium foods such as bananas, oranges, potatoes, and tomatoes.
- **Choose Low-Potassium Alternatives:** Opt for apples, berries, grapes, cauliflower, and bell peppers instead.
- **Read Food Labels:** Check for potassium content, especially in processed foods and beverages.
- **Consult Your Doctor:** Regularly check your blood potassium levels and follow dietary advice from your healthcare provider.

By effectively managing potassium intake, you can help prevent complications and support overall heart health.

Hydration and Fluid Management

6.1 Understanding Fluid Needs

Understanding fluid needs is essential for managing Stage 3 kidney disease. Proper hydration supports overall health, but it's crucial to balance fluid intake to avoid overloading the kidneys. Here are some key points:

- **Consult Your Doctor:** Get personalized advice on the appropriate amount of fluid intake based on your condition.
- **Monitor Fluid Intake:** Keep track of all fluids consumed, including water, beverages, and foods with high water content like soups and fruits.
- **Control Portions:** Use smaller cups and limit high-fluid foods if necessary to avoid excessive intake.
- **Balance Hydration:** Ensure you're drinking enough to stay hydrated without causing fluid retention or swelling.

By understanding and managing your fluid needs, you can help maintain kidney function and prevent complications.

6.2 Beverages to Avoid and Prefer

Choosing the right beverages is crucial for managing Stage 3 kidney disease. Here are some guidelines:

Beverages to Avoid:

- **Sodas and Colas:** High in phosphorus and sugars.
- **Sports and Energy Drinks:** Often contain high potassium and phosphorus.
- **Alcohol:** Can affect kidney function and blood pressure.
- **Caffeinated Beverages:** Limit intake, as excessive caffeine can cause dehydration.

Beverages to Prefer:

- **Water:** The best choice for hydration.
- **Herbal Teas:** Low in phosphorus and caffeine-free.
- **Clear Broths:** Low-sodium options can be hydrating.
- **Specialty Kidney-Friendly Drinks:** Designed to meet specific dietary needs.

Opting for the right beverages can help manage your kidney health effectively.

Grocery Shopping and Pantry Essentials

7.1 Kidney-Friendly Grocery List

Creating a kidney-friendly grocery list helps ensure you have the right ingredients to manage Stage 3 kidney disease effectively. Focus on foods that support kidney health while adhering to dietary restrictions. Here's a guide for a kidney-friendly grocery list:

Fruits:

- Apples
- Berries (blueberries, strawberries, raspberries)
- Grapes
- Pineapple
- Pears

Vegetables:

- Bell peppers
- Cauliflower
- Cucumbers
- Green beans
- Lettuce
- Zucchini

Proteins:

- Chicken breast
- Turkey
- Fish (such as salmon and tilapia)
- Egg whites

- Tofu

Grains:

- Brown rice
- Quinoa
- Whole wheat bread (low-sodium)
- Oats

Dairy Alternatives:

- Almond milk
- Rice milk
- Low-phosphorus yogurt (if advised)

Healthy Fats:

- Olive oil
- Avocados
- Unsalted nuts (in moderation)

Miscellaneous:

- Low-sodium broth
- Fresh herbs and spices (for flavoring)
- Whole-grain pasta (in moderation)

Beverages:

- Water
- Herbal teas (like chamomile or peppermint)

By selecting these kidney-friendly options, you can support your health and manage your dietary needs effectively.

7.2 Stocking a Renal-Friendly Pantry

Stocking a renal-friendly pantry involves choosing ingredients that support kidney health while adhering to dietary restrictions for Stage 3 kidney disease. Here's how to build and maintain a kidney-friendly pantry:

1. Choose Low-Sodium Options:

- **Canned Goods:** Select low-sodium or no-salt-added versions of canned vegetables, beans, and soups.
- **Broths:** Opt for low-sodium vegetable or chicken broths for cooking and flavoring.

2. Include Low-Potassium Foods:

- **Grains:** Stock up on low-potassium grains like quinoa, brown rice, and whole wheat pasta.
- **Baking Supplies:** Use low-potassium flours and sugar substitutes if needed.

3. Incorporate Low-Phosphorus Items:

- **Condiments:** Choose low-phosphorus condiments and sauces, avoiding those with added phosphates.
- **Snacks:** Opt for unsalted popcorn, rice cakes, and whole-grain crackers in moderation.

4. Select Healthy Fats:

- **Oils:** Keep olive oil and canola oil on hand for cooking and dressings.
- **Nut Butters:** Choose unsalted varieties of almond or cashew butter, using them sparingly.

5. Stock Fresh Herbs and Spices:

- **Herbs:** Basil, parsley, cilantro, and rosemary can add flavor without added sodium.
- **Spices:** Use spices like turmeric, paprika, and garlic powder to enhance flavor in your meals.

6. Manage Fluids and Beverages:

- **Water:** Save a lot of water close by for hydration.
- **Herbal Teas:** Stock caffeine-free herbal teas for variety in your fluid intake.

7. Plan for Convenience:

- **Frozen Vegetables:** Opt for frozen vegetables without added sauces or sodium.
- **Prepared Meals:** If needed, have kidney-friendly prepared meal options for convenience.

8. Monitor Expiration Dates:

- Regularly check expiration dates and rotate pantry items to ensure freshness and avoid waste.

By thoughtfully stocking your pantry with these items, you can create a convenient and supportive environment for managing Stage 3 kidney disease, ensuring that your dietary needs are met with ease.

Breakfast Recipes

8.2.1 Blueberry Oatmeal

Ingredients

- **Oats**: 1 cup (old-fashioned or quick oats)
- **Milk**: 2 ½ cups (any type, such as almond, oat, or regular)
- **Blueberries**: 2 cups (fresh)
- **Honey**: 2 tablespoons (plus more for topping)
- **Salt**: a pinch
- **Cinnamon**: ¼ teaspoon (optional)
- **Chia seeds**: ½ tablespoon (optional for added nutrition)
- **Maple syrup**: 1 teaspoon (optional for sweetness)

Directions

1. **Blend Blueberries**: In a blender, combine 1 ½ cups of blueberries with the milk and blend until smooth. Reserve the remaining ½ cup of blueberries for topping later.
2. **Cook Oatmeal**: In a medium saucepan, combine the blueberry-milk mixture, oats, salt, and honey. Bring to a boil over medium heat, stirring occasionally.
3. **Simmer**: Once boiling, reduce the heat to low and continue stirring for about 5-7 minutes, or until the oatmeal reaches your desired consistency. If you want to incorporate chia seeds, add them during this step.
4. **Serve**: Pour the oatmeal into bowls and top with the reserved blueberries, a drizzle of honey, and any additional toppings you prefer (like nuts or more fruit).

Cooking and Prep Time

- **Prep Time**: 5 minutes
- **Cook Time**: 5-7 minutes
- **Total Time**: Approximately 10-12 minutes

Serving

This recipe serves about 2 bowls of oatmeal, making it perfect for sharing or meal prep.

Nutrition Information (per serving)

- **Calories**: Approximately 303 kcal
- **Carbohydrates**: 48 g
- **Protein**: 9 g
- **Fat**: 8 g
- **Saturated Fat**: 1 g
- **Fiber**: 8 g
- **Sugar**: 11 g
- **Sodium**: 324 mg
- **Potassium**: 424 mg

8.2.2 Spinach and Mushroom Egg White Omelette

Ingredients

- **Egg Whites**: 6 large egg whites
- **Mushrooms**: 6 medium mushrooms, sliced
- **Spinach**: 1/2 cup fresh spinach leaves, stems removed
- **Cheese**: 1/2 cup Colby Jack cheese, finely shredded
- **Olive Oil**: 1 tbsp
- **Butter**: 2 tsp unsalted butter
- **Salt and Pepper**: to taste

Directions

1. **Sauté Mushrooms**: Heat a skillet over medium heat and add 1 tbsp olive oil. Sauté the sliced mushrooms until golden brown and soft, about 4-5 minutes. Season lightly with salt and pepper. Remove from heat and set aside.
2. **Whisk Egg Whites**: In a small bowl, whisk the egg whites until frothy and well combined.
3. **Cook Omelette**: Heat a 10-inch nonstick pan over medium heat and coat the bottom with 1 tsp butter. Pour in half of the whisked egg whites, enough to cover the pan in a thin layer. Let cook for 2 minutes or until the bottom is starting to set.
4. **Flip and Fill**: Use a spatula to gently flip the egg white layer over. Immediately sprinkle 1/4 of the shredded cheese over the surface. Place the sautéed mushrooms on one half of the omelette and the fresh spinach leaves on the other half.
5. **Fold and Serve**: Use the spatula to fold the omelette in half, being careful not to deflate the fluffy eggs. Slide the folded omelette onto a plate. Repeat steps 3 and 4 to make a second omelette. Top with the remaining cheese, salt, and pepper to taste.

Cooking and Prep Time

- **Prep Time**: 5 minutes
- **Cook Time**: 10 minutes
- **Total Time**: 15 minutes

Serving

This recipe makes two omelettes, perfect for sharing or enjoying one now and saving the other for later.

Nutrition Information (per serving)

- **Calories**: 206
- **Protein**: 25g
- **Fat**: 10g
- **Carbohydrates**: 4g
- **Fiber**: 1g
- **Sugar**: 2g
- **Cholesterol**: 10mg
- **Sodium**: 416mg

8.2.3 Low-Phosphorus Pancakes

Ingredients

- **Rice Milk**: ½ cup (or Coffeerich® milk substitute)
- **All-Purpose Flour**: ½ cup
- **Egg**: 1 large
- **Sugar**: 1 tsp (or Splenda® for a sugar substitute)
- **Vegetable Oil**: 1 tbsp
- **Non-Hydrogenated Margarine**: for cooking

Directions

1. **Mix Ingredients**: In a mixing bowl, combine the rice milk, flour, egg, sugar, and vegetable oil. Stir until the mixture is smooth and well combined.
2. **Heat Skillet**: Heat a skillet over medium heat and melt enough non-hydrogenated margarine to coat the bottom.
3. **Cook Pancakes**: Pour about ¼ cup of the batter into the skillet. Gently tilt the skillet to spread the batter evenly. Cook for about 1 minute, or until the edges start to turn golden.
4. **Flip and Finish**: Use a spatula to flip the pancake and cook the other side until golden brown, about another minute.
5. **Repeat**: Continue cooking the remaining batter, adding more margarine to the skillet as needed.

Cooking and Prep Time

- **Prep Time**: 5 minutes
- **Cook Time**: 10 minutes
- **Total Time**: 15 minutes

Serving

This recipe yields approximately 4 pancakes, with each pancake serving as one portion.
Nutrition Information (per pancake)

- **Calories**: Approximately 100 kcal
- **Protein**: 2 g
- **Carbohydrates**: 15 g
- **Fat**: 4 g
- **Saturated Fat**: 1 g
- **Sugar**: 1 g
- **Sodium**: 50 mg
- **Phosphorus**: Approximately 30 mg

8.2.4 Apple Cinnamon Quinoa

Ingredients

- **Quinoa**: ½ cup uncooked quinoa, rinsed
- **Apple**: 1 medium apple, cored, peeled, and chopped
- **Almond Milk**: 1½ cups unsweetened almond milk (or any dairy-free milk)
- **Maple Syrup**: 1 tablespoon (optional, for added sweetness)
- **Cinnamon**: 1 teaspoon ground cinnamon
- **Vanilla Extract**: ½ teaspoon (optional)
- **Salt**: a pinch
- **Raisins**: ¼ cup (optional, for added sweetness and texture)

Directions

1. **Rinse Quinoa**: Rinse the quinoa under cold water in a fine mesh strainer to remove any bitterness.
2. **Combine Ingredients**: In a medium saucepan, combine the rinsed quinoa, chopped apple, almond milk, maple syrup, cinnamon, vanilla extract, salt, and raisins (if using).
3. **Cook**: Bring the mixture to a boil over medium-high heat. Once boiling, reduce the heat to low, cover the saucepan, and let it simmer for about 15-20 minutes, or until the quinoa is tender and has absorbed most of the liquid.
4. **Rest**: Remove the saucepan from heat and let it sit, covered, for an additional 5 minutes. This allows the quinoa to steam and become fluffy.
5. **Serve**: Fluff the quinoa with a fork and serve warm. You can top it with additional apple slices, a drizzle of maple syrup, or nuts if desired.

Cooking and Prep Time

- **Prep Time**: 5 minutes
- **Cook Time**: 20 minutes
- **Total Time**: 25 minutes

Serving

This recipe serves about 2 portions, making it ideal for a cozy breakfast for two.

Nutrition Information (per serving)

- **Calories**: Approximately 220 kcal
- **Protein**: 6 g
- **Fat**: 3 g
- **Carbohydrates**: 42 g
- **Fiber**: 5 g
- **Sugar**: 8 g
- **Sodium**: 50 mg
- **Potassium**: 350 mg

8.2.5 Kidney-Friendly Smoothie

Ingredients

- **Unsweetened Plant Milk**: 1 cup (check ingredient list for phosphorus additives)
- **Unsweetened Plant Yogurt**: 1/4 cup (check ingredient list for phosphorus additives)
- **Ground Flaxseed**: 1 Tbsp
- **Chia Seeds**: 1 Tbsp
- **Raw Leafy Greens**: 1 cup (spinach, arugula, or kale)
- **Frozen Pineapple**: 1 cup
- **Frozen Blueberries**: 1/2 cup (or mixed berries)

Directions

1. **Combine Ingredients**: In a blender, add the plant milk, plant yogurt, ground flaxseed, chia seeds, leafy greens, frozen pineapple, and frozen blueberries.
2. **Blend**: Blend all the ingredients until smooth and creamy.
3. **Serve**: Pour the smoothie into a glass and enjoy immediately.

Prep Time

5 minutes

Serving

This recipe makes 1 serving.

Nutrition Information (per smoothie)

- **Calories**: 301
- **Protein**: 7.5 g
- **Carbohydrates**: 45 g
- **Fiber**: 12 g
- **Potassium**: 513 mg
- **Phosphorus**: 140 mg

8.2.6 Banana Nut Muffins

Ingredients

- **Ripe Bananas**: 3 medium (about 1 ½ cups mashed)
- **All-Purpose Flour**: 1 ½ cups
- **Granulated Sugar**: ½ cup
- **Light Brown Sugar**: ¼ cup, packed
- **Baking Soda**: 1 teaspoon
- **Baking Powder**: 1 teaspoon
- **Salt**: ½ teaspoon
- **Ground Cinnamon**: ¾ teaspoon
- **Large Egg**: 1
- **Vegetable Oil**: ⅓ cup
- **Vanilla Extract**: 1 ½ teaspoons
- **Chopped Pecans or Walnuts**: 1 cup
- **Coarse Sugar**: for topping (optional)

Directions

1. **Preheat Oven**: Preheat your oven to 425°F (220°C). Grease a muffin tin or line it with muffin liners.
2. **Mix Dry Ingredients**: In a large mixing bowl, whisk together the flour, baking soda, baking powder, salt, and cinnamon.
3. **Combine Wet Ingredients**: In another bowl, mash the bananas until smooth. Then, mix in the granulated sugar, brown sugar, egg, vegetable oil, and vanilla extract until well combined.
4. **Combine Mixtures**: Pour the banana mixture into the dry ingredients and stir gently until just combined. Do not overmix. Fold in the chopped nuts.
5. **Fill Muffin Cups**: Evenly scoop the batter into the prepared muffin cups, filling each about ¾ full. If desired, sprinkle coarse sugar on top for added crunch.

6. **Bake**: Bake in the preheated oven for 8 minutes. Without opening the oven door, reduce the temperature to 350°F (175°C) and continue baking for another 6-8 minutes, or until a toothpick inserted into the center comes out clean.
7. **Cool**: Let the muffins cool in the pan for a few minutes before transferring them to a wire rack to cool completely.

Prep Time

- **Prep Time**: 15 minutes
- **Cook Time**: 15 minutes
- **Total Time**: 30 minutes

Serving

This recipe yields approximately 12 muffins.

Nutrition Information (per muffin)

- **Calories**: Approximately 150 kcal
- **Protein**: 3 g
- **Fat**: 5 g
- **Carbohydrates**: 24 g
- **Fiber**: 1 g
- **Sugar**: 8 g
- **Sodium**: 100 mg

8.2.7 Scrambled Tofu with Veggies

Ingredients

- **Firm or Extra-Firm Tofu**: 1 block (14-16 oz), drained and crumbled
- **Olive Oil**: 1 tbsp
- **Onion**: 1 small, diced
- **Bell Pepper**: 1 medium, diced
- **Mushrooms**: 6-8 medium, sliced
- **Spinach**: 2 cups fresh, chopped
- **Turmeric**: 1 tsp
- **Garlic Powder**: 1/2 tsp
- **Onion Powder**: 1/2 tsp
- **Nutritional Yeast**: 2 tbsp
- **Salt and Pepper**: to taste

Directions

1. **Crumble Tofu**: In a large skillet over medium heat, crumble the tofu into bite-sized pieces using your hands or a fork.
2. **Sauté Veggies**: Add the olive oil to the skillet and sauté the onion, bell pepper, and mushrooms until softened, about 5-7 minutes.
3. **Add Tofu and Seasonings**: Stir in the crumbled tofu, turmeric, garlic powder, onion powder, and nutritional yeast. Cook for 2-3 minutes, stirring frequently.
4. **Add Spinach**: Add the chopped spinach to the skillet and cook until wilted, about 1-2 minutes.
5. **Season to Taste**: Season with salt and pepper to your liking.

Cooking and Prep Time

- **Prep Time**: 10 minutes
- **Cook Time**: 10-12 minutes
- **Total Time**: 20-22 minutes

Serving

This recipe serves approximately 2-3 people, depending on portion size.

Nutrition Information (per serving)

- **Calories**: Approximately 250 kcal
- **Protein**: 20 g
- **Fat**: 12 g
- **Carbohydrates**: 16 g
- **Fiber**: 5 g
- **Sugar**: 4 g
- **Sodium**: 500 mg

8.2.8 Berry Parfait with Greek Yogurt

Ingredients

- **Greek Yogurt**: 2 cups plain or vanilla
- **Honey**: 2 tablespoons (optional, for sweetening yogurt)
- **Mixed Berries**: 2 cups (such as blueberries, raspberries, and blackberries)
- **Granola**: 1 cup of your favorite variety
- **Chia Seeds**: 1 tablespoon (optional)

Directions

1. **Sweeten Yogurt**: If using plain Greek yogurt, mix in the honey until well combined. Vanilla yogurt can be used without additional sweetening.
2. **Layer Parfait**: In a glass or jar, layer the ingredients in the following order: 1/3 of the yogurt, 1/3 of the berries, and 1/3 of the granola. Repeat the layers two more times, ending with granola on top.
3. **Refrigerate**: Cover and refrigerate the parfait until ready to serve, or enjoy immediately.
4. **Serve**: Top with a sprinkle of chia seeds (if using) and an extra drizzle of honey, if desired.

Prep Time

- **Prep Time**: 5 minutes
- **Total Time**: 5 minutes

Serving

This recipe makes 2 servings, perfect for sharing or enjoying one now and saving the other for later.

Nutrition Information (per serving)

- **Calories**: Approximately 300 kcal
- **Protein**: 18 g
- **Fat**: 3 g

- **Carbohydrates**: 50 g
- **Fiber**: 7 g
- **Sugar**: 25 g
- **Sodium**: 65 mg

8.2.9 Sweet Potato Hash

Ingredients

- **Sweet Potatoes**: 2 large, peeled and diced into ½-inch cubes
- **Olive Oil**: 2 tablespoons
- **Red Onion**: ½ medium, diced
- **Poblano Pepper**: 1, stemmed, seeded, and chopped (or substitute with bell pepper)
- **Garlic**: 2 cloves, thinly sliced
- **Chili Powder**: 1 teaspoon
- **Lacinato Kale**: 4 leaves, stemmed and torn (or substitute with spinach)
- **Eggs**: 4 large (optional for topping)
- **Salt and Pepper**: to taste
- **Avocado**: 1, sliced (for serving)
- **Fresh Cilantro**: for garnish (optional)
- **Hot Sauce**: for serving (optional)
- **Lime Wedges**: for squeezing (optional)

Directions

1. **Sauté Vegetables**: In a large skillet, heat the olive oil over medium heat. Add the diced onion and poblano pepper, cooking until softened, about 5-7 minutes. Add the sliced garlic and cook for an additional minute until fragrant.
2. **Cook Sweet Potatoes**: Add the diced sweet potatoes to the skillet. Stir to combine and cook for about 10 minutes, stirring occasionally, until they start to soften.
3. **Season**: Sprinkle in the chili powder, salt, and pepper. Stir well to coat the sweet potatoes with the spices.
4. **Add Greens**: Fold in the torn kale and cook until it wilts, about 2-3 minutes.

5. **Optional Eggs**: If using eggs, create four wells in the hash and crack an egg into each well. Cover the skillet and cook for 3-5 minutes, or until the eggs are set to your liking.
6. **Serve**: Serve the sweet potato hash warm, topped with sliced avocado, fresh cilantro, and hot sauce if desired. Squeeze lime juice over the top for added flavor.

Cooking and Prep Time

- **Prep Time**: 10 minutes
- **Cook Time**: 20 minutes
- **Total Time**: 30 minutes

Serving

This recipe serves approximately 4 people.

Nutrition Information (per serving without eggs)

- **Calories**: Approximately 220 kcal
- **Protein**: 4 g
- **Fat**: 10 g
- **Carbohydrates**: 30 g
- **Fiber**: 5 g
- **Sugar**: 5 g
- **Sodium**: 300 mg

8.2.10 Avocado Toast

Ingredients

- **Bread**: 2 slices of your choice (whole grain, sourdough, or gluten-free)
- **Avocado**: 1 ripe avocado, pitted and mashed
- **Olive Oil**: 1 tsp
- **Lemon Juice**: 1 tbsp
- **Salt and Pepper**: to taste
- **Toppings (optional)**:
    - Spinach, sautéed
    - Cherry tomatoes, halved
    - Sliced mushrooms, sautéed
    - Fried egg
    - Everything Bagel Seasoning

Directions

1. **Toast the bread**: Toast the bread slices until golden brown.
2. **Mash the avocado**: In a small bowl, mash the avocado with a fork until slightly chunky. Add olive oil, lemon juice, salt, and pepper. Mix well.
3. **Assemble the toast**: Spread the mashed avocado mixture evenly over the toasted bread slices.
4. **Add toppings (optional)**: Top the avocado toast with your desired toppings, such as sautéed spinach, cherry tomatoes, sliced mushrooms, a fried egg, or a sprinkle of Everything Bagel Seasoning.

Cooking and Prep Time

- **Prep Time**: 5 minutes
- **Cook Time**: 5 minutes (if adding toppings)
- **Total Time**: 10 minutes

Serving

This recipe makes 2 slices of avocado toast.

Nutrition Information (per serving without toppings)

- **Calories**: Approximately 250 kcal
- **Protein**: 5 g
- **Fat**: 15 g
- **Carbohydrates**: 25 g
- **Fiber**: 10 g
- **Sugar**: 2 g
- **Sodium**: 300 mg

8.2.11 Whole Grain Waffles

Ingredients

- **Whole Wheat Flour**: 2 cups (260g)
- **Baking Powder**: 1 tablespoon
- **Ground Cinnamon**: 1/2 teaspoon
- **Salt**: 1/4 teaspoon
- **Unsalted Butter**: 6 tablespoons (85g), melted and slightly cooled
- **Eggs**: 2 large, at room temperature
- **Brown Sugar**: 2 tablespoons (25g), packed
- **Buttermilk**: 1 3/4 cups (420ml)
- **Vanilla Extract**: 1 teaspoon

Directions

1. **Preheat Waffle Iron**: Preheat your waffle iron according to the manufacturer's instructions.
2. **Mix Dry Ingredients**: In a large bowl, whisk together the whole wheat flour, baking powder, cinnamon, and salt.
3. **Mix Wet Ingredients**: In another bowl, whisk together the melted butter, eggs, brown sugar, buttermilk, and vanilla extract until well combined.
4. **Combine Mixtures**: Pour the wet ingredients into the dry ingredients and stir gently until just combined. Avoid overmixing; it's okay if there are a few lumps.
5. **Cook Waffles**: Grease the preheated waffle iron if necessary. Pour about 1/3 cup of batter into each section of the waffle iron (adjust based on the size of your iron). Close the lid and cook according to the manufacturer's instructions, typically for about 4-5 minutes, or until the waffles are golden brown.
6. **Serve**: Serve the waffles warm with your favorite toppings such as fresh fruit, maple syrup, yogurt, or nut butter.

Cooking and Prep Time

- **Prep Time**: 10 minutes
- **Cook Time**: 15 minutes (includes batches)
- **Total Time**: 25 minutes

Serving

This recipe yields approximately 6-8 waffles, depending on the size of your waffle iron.

Nutrition Information (per waffle without toppings)

- **Calories**: Approximately 150 kcal
- **Protein**: 5 g
- **Fat**: 7 g
- **Carbohydrates**: 20 g
- **Fiber**: 3 g
- **Sugar**: 2 g
- **Sodium**: 200 mg

8.2.12 Pumpkin Spice Overnight Oats

Ingredients

- **Rolled Oats**: 1/2 cup
- **Unsweetened Almond Milk**: 1 cup
- **Pumpkin Puree**: 1/4 cup
- **Maple Syrup**: 1 tablespoon (or honey)
- **Chia Seeds**: 1 tablespoon
- **Pumpkin Pie Spice**: 1/2 teaspoon
- **Cinnamon**: 1/4 teaspoon
- **Vanilla Extract**: 1/4 teaspoon
- **Pinch of Salt**

Directions

1. **In a jar or bowl with a lid**, combine the rolled oats, almond milk, pumpkin puree, maple syrup, chia seeds, pumpkin pie spice, cinnamon, vanilla extract, and a pinch of salt. Stir well to combine.
2. **Cover and refrigerate overnight or for at least 4 hours.** The oats will thicken as they absorb the liquid.
3. **In the morning**, give the overnight oats a stir. You can enjoy them chilled or warm them up in the microwave for 30-60 seconds.
4. **Top with your favorite toppings**, such as sliced bananas, chopped nuts, a drizzle of nut butter, or a sprinkle of extra cinnamon or pumpkin pie spice.

Prep Time

5 minutes

Serving

This recipe makes one serving. Double or triple the ingredients to make multiple servings at once.

Nutrition Information (per serving)

- **Calories**: 300
- **Protein**: 8g
- **Fat**: 9g
- **Carbohydrates**: 48g
- **Fiber**: 9g
- **Sugar**: 12g

8.2.13 Low-Sodium Breakfast Burrito

Ingredients

- **Turkey Sausage**: 1 lb, casings removed
- **Olive Oil**: 1 tbsp
- **Onion**: 1 small, diced
- **Bell Peppers**: 1 red and 1 green, diced
- **Eggs**: 12 large
- **Egg Whites**: 6 large
- **Black Beans**: 1 (15 oz) can, rinsed and drained
- **Spinach**: 2 cups, chopped
- **Low-Sodium Cheese**: 1 cup, shredded (such as mozzarella or cheddar)
- **Low-Sodium Tortillas**: 6 (10-inch), whole wheat or low-carb

Directions

1. In a large skillet over medium heat, cook the turkey sausage, breaking it up with a wooden spoon as it cooks, until no longer pink, about 5-7 minutes. Transfer to a plate and set aside.
2. In the same skillet, heat the olive oil over medium heat. Add the onion and bell peppers and cook until softened, about 5 minutes.
3. In a large bowl, whisk together the eggs, egg whites, and a pinch of black pepper. Pour the egg mixture into the skillet with the vegetables and cook, stirring occasionally, until the eggs are scrambled and cooked through, about 5 minutes.
4. Stir in the black beans, spinach, and cooked turkey sausage. Remove from heat.
5. Warm the tortillas according to package instructions.
6. Divide the egg mixture evenly among the tortillas, leaving a 1-inch border. Top each with 2-3 tbsp of shredded cheese.
7. Fold the bottom of each tortilla up over the filling, then fold in the sides and continue rolling up tightly into a burrito.
8. Wrap each burrito in foil or parchment paper and freeze for up to 3 months.

Cooking and Prep Time

- **Prep Time**: 15 minutes
- **Cook Time**: 20 minutes
- **Total Time**: 35 minutes

Serving

This recipe makes 6 burritos.

Nutrition Information (per burrito)

- **Calories**: 350
- **Protein**: 28g
- **Fat**: 12g
- **Carbohydrates**: 35g
- **Fiber**: 7g
- **Sodium**: 350mg

8.2.14 Almond Butter and Banana Toast

Ingredients

- **Whole Grain Bread**: 2 slices
- **Almond Butter**: 2-3 tablespoons
- **Banana**: 1 medium, sliced
- **Cinnamon**: 1/4 teaspoon (optional)
- **Honey**: 1 teaspoon (optional)

Directions

1. **Toast the bread** until golden brown.
2. **Spread the almond butter** evenly over the toasted bread slices.
3. **Arrange the banana slices** on top of the almond butter.
4. **Sprinkle with cinnamon** and drizzle with honey if desired.

Prep Time

5 minutes

Cooking Time

2-3 minutes for toasting the bread

Serving

This recipe makes 2 slices of almond butter and banana toast.

Nutrition Information (per serving)

- **Calories**: Approximately 300
- **Protein**: 8 g
- **Fat**: 15 g
- **Carbohydrates**: 35 g
- **Fiber**: 6 g
- **Sugar**: 12 g
- **Sodium**: 200 mg

8.2.15 Lemon Poppy Seed Muffins

Ingredients

- **All-Purpose Flour**: 1 ½ cups
- **Granulated Sugar**: ¾ cup
- **Baking Powder**: 2 teaspoons
- **Baking Soda**: ½ teaspoon
- **Salt**: ¼ teaspoon
- **Poppy Seeds**: 2 tablespoons
- **Lemon Zest**: 1 tablespoon (from about 1 lemon)
- **Eggs**: 2 large
- **Buttermilk**: ½ cup (or milk with 1 teaspoon vinegar added)
- **Vegetable Oil**: ⅓ cup
- **Lemon Juice**: 2 tablespoons (freshly squeezed)
- **Vanilla Extract**: 1 teaspoon

Directions

1. **Preheat Oven**: Preheat your oven to 350°F (175°C). Line a muffin tin with paper liners or grease it lightly.
2. **Mix Dry Ingredients**: In a large bowl, whisk together the flour, sugar, baking powder, baking soda, salt, poppy seeds, and lemon zest until well combined.
3. **Mix Wet Ingredients**: In another bowl, whisk together the eggs, buttermilk, vegetable oil, lemon juice, and vanilla extract until smooth.
4. **Combine Mixtures**: Pour the wet ingredients into the dry ingredients and stir gently until just combined. Be careful not to overmix; a few lumps are okay.
5. **Fill Muffin Tin**: Divide the batter evenly among the prepared muffin cups, filling each about ¾ full.
6. **Bake**: Bake in the preheated oven for 18-20 minutes, or until a toothpick inserted into the center comes out clean.

7. **Cool**: Allow the muffins to cool in the pan for 5 minutes before transferring them to a wire rack to cool completely.

Cooking and Prep Time

- **Prep Time**: 10 minutes
- **Cook Time**: 20 minutes
- **Total Time**: 30 minutes

Serving

This recipe yields approximately 12 muffins.

Nutrition Information (per muffin)

- **Calories**: Approximately 180 kcal
- **Protein**: 3 g
- **Fat**: 7 g
- **Carbohydrates**: 27 g
- **Fiber**: 1 g
- **Sugar**: 10 g
- **Sodium**: 150 mg

Lunch Recipes

9.2.1 Grilled Chicken Salad

Ingredients

- 1 lb boneless skinless chicken breasts
- 6 cups chopped romaine lettuce
- 3/4 cup halved cherry tomatoes
- 3/4 cup corn kernels
- 3/4 cup chopped cucumber
- 1/4 cup thinly sliced red onion
- 1/2 cup cooked crumbled bacon (optional)
- 1/2 cup crumbled blue cheese (optional)
- 1 avocado, sliced

Dressing:

- 3 tbsp lemon juice
- 2 tbsp Dijon mustard
- 3 tbsp red wine vinegar
- 2 tsp sugar
- 2 tbsp minced shallot
- 1/2 tsp dried oregano
- 1 1/2 tsp dried parsley
- 2/3 cup olive oil
- Salt and pepper to taste

Directions

1. Make the dressing by whisking together the lemon juice, mustard, vinegar, sugar, shallot, oregano, parsley, olive oil, salt and pepper. Set aside half the dressing.

2. Add the chicken to the remaining dressing and marinate for 1-8 hours in the fridge.
3. Grill the chicken for 5-6 minutes per side until it reaches 165°F. Let rest 5 minutes before slicing.
4. In a large bowl, toss the romaine with half the reserved dressing.
5. Top with the sliced grilled chicken, tomatoes, corn, cucumber, onion, bacon, blue cheese and avocado.
6. Drizzle with the remaining dressing and serve.

Cooking and Prep Time

- **Prep Time:** 20 minutes (plus marinating time)
- **Cooking Time:** 12 minutes
- **Total Time:** Approximately 1 hour (including marinating)

Serving Suggestions

This salad serves 4 and pairs well with crusty bread or a light soup for a complete meal.

Nutritional Information (per serving)

- **Calories:** Approximately 450-500 (depending on added ingredients)
- **Protein:** 30-35g
- **Fat:** 30g (includes healthy fats from olive oil and avocado)
- **Carbohydrates:** 15-20g
- **Fiber:** 5-7g

9.2.2 Quinoa and Black Bean Salad

Ingredients

- 1 cup uncooked quinoa, rinsed
- 1 (15 oz) can black beans, drained and rinsed
- 1 1/2 cups diced English cucumber
- 1 bell pepper (red, yellow or orange), diced
- 1 cup diced carrot (about 2 medium)
- 1/4 cup sliced green onions (white and light green parts only)
- 1/4 cup chopped cilantro

For the Dressing:

- 1/4 cup olive oil
- 1/4 cup freshly squeezed lime juice (about 2 limes)
- 1 tsp ground cumin
- 1 tsp fine sea salt
- 1/8 tsp ground cayenne pepper (or to taste)

Directions

1. **Cook the quinoa:** In a medium saucepan, combine the rinsed quinoa and 2 cups water or stock. Bring to a boil, then reduce heat to low, cover and simmer for 15 minutes until quinoa is tender and liquid is absorbed. Fluff with a fork and let cool slightly.
2. **Make the dressing:** In a small bowl or jar, whisk together the olive oil, lime juice, cumin, salt and cayenne.
3. **Assemble the salad:** In a large bowl, combine the cooked quinoa, black beans, cucumber, bell pepper, carrot, green onions and cilantro. Pour the dressing over top and stir gently until well coated.
4. **Chill and serve:** For best flavor, let the salad chill in the fridge for 30 minutes before serving to allow the flavors to blend. Serve chilled or at room temperature.

Cooking and Prep Time

- **Prep Time:** 20 minutes
- **Cook Time:** 15 minutes
- **Total Time:** 35 minutes

Serving and Nutrition

This recipe makes about 6 servings. Per serving:

- **Calories:** 262
- **Protein:** 8g
- **Fat:** 12g
- **Carbs:** 34g
- **Fiber:** 7g

9.2.3 Turkey and Avocado Wrap

Ingredients

- 4 large tortillas or wraps (10-12 inches)
- 1 ripe avocado
- 2 tbsp mayonnaise or Greek yogurt
- 1 tbsp fresh lime juice
- Salt and pepper to taste
- 8 oz thinly sliced deli turkey
- 2 cups shredded romaine lettuce
- 1 cup halved cherry tomatoes
- 1 cup thinly sliced cucumber
- 1/2 cup thinly sliced red onion (optional)

Instructions

1. In a small bowl, mash the avocado with the mayonnaise or yogurt, lime juice, salt and pepper until well combined into a creamy spread.
2. Lay the tortillas out flat. Spread 2-3 tbsp of the avocado mixture evenly over each tortilla, leaving a 1-inch border.
3. Layer each tortilla with 2 oz turkey, 1/2 cup lettuce, 1/4 cup tomatoes, 1/4 cup cucumbers and 2 tbsp red onion (if using).
4. Fold the bottom of the tortilla up over the filling, fold in both sides and then continue rolling up tightly into a wrap.
5. Slice each wrap in half diagonally and serve immediately or refrigerate until ready to eat.

Cooking and Prep Time

- Prep Time: 10 minutes
- Total Time: 10 minutes

Serving

This recipe makes 4 wraps, serving 2 people as a main dish or 4 people as a lighter lunch or snack.

Nutrition (per serving)

- Calories: 350
- Protein: 20g
- Fat: 18g
- Carbs: 32g
- Fiber: 6g

9.2.4 Lentil Soup

Ingredients

- ¼ cup extra virgin olive oil
- 1 medium yellow or white onion, chopped
- 2 carrots, peeled and chopped
- 4 garlic cloves, minced
- 2 teaspoons ground cumin
- 1 teaspoon curry powder
- ½ teaspoon dried thyme
- 1 (28 oz) can diced tomatoes, lightly drained
- 1 cup brown or green lentils, rinsed
- 4 cups vegetable broth
- 2 cups water
- 1 teaspoon salt (more to taste)
- Pinch of red pepper flakes
- Freshly ground black pepper, to taste
- 1 cup chopped kale or collard greens
- 1 to 2 tablespoons lemon juice (to taste)

Directions

1. **Sauté Vegetables:** In a large pot, heat the olive oil over medium heat. Add the chopped onion and carrots, cooking until the onion is translucent (about 5 minutes).
2. **Add Spices and Garlic:** Stir in the minced garlic, cumin, curry powder, and thyme. Cook for another 30 seconds until fragrant.
3. **Add Tomatoes and Lentils:** Pour in the drained diced tomatoes, lentils, vegetable broth, water, salt, and red pepper flakes. Season with black pepper. Bring to a boil.

4. **Simmer:** Reduce the heat to a gentle simmer, cover partially, and cook for 25-30 minutes until the lentils are tender.
5. **Blend (optional):** For a creamier texture, blend about 2 cups of the soup in a blender or use an immersion blender to puree a portion of the soup. Return it to the pot.
6. **Add Greens:** Stir in the chopped kale or collard greens and cook for an additional 5 minutes until the greens are tender.
7. **Finish with Lemon:** Remove from heat and stir in lemon juice. Adjust seasoning with more salt, pepper, or lemon juice as desired.
8. **Serve:** Ladle the soup into bowls and enjoy hot.

Cooking and Prep Time

- **Prep Time:** 10 minutes
- **Cook Time:** 45 minutes
- **Total Time:** 55 minutes

Serving

This recipe yields about 4 servings.

Nutrition (per serving)

- **Calories:** Approximately 300
- **Protein:** 15g
- **Fat:** 10g
- **Carbohydrates:** 40g
- **Fiber:** 15g

9.2.5 Tuna Salad with Olive Oil Dressing

Ingredients

For the Salad:

- 3 (5 oz) cans chunk light tuna in water, drained
- 1 cup chopped romaine lettuce
- 1/2 cup halved cherry tomatoes
- 1/2 cup chopped cucumber
- 1/4 cup thinly sliced red onion
- 2 tbsp chopped fresh parsley
- 2 tbsp chopped fresh basil

For the Dressing:

- 3 tbsp olive oil
- 2 tbsp lemon juice
- 1 tbsp Dijon mustard
- 1 tsp dried oregano
- 1/4 tsp red pepper flakes (optional)
- Salt and pepper to taste

Instructions

1. In a medium bowl, break up the drained tuna with a fork into flaky chunks.
2. Add the chopped romaine, tomatoes, cucumber, red onion, parsley and basil. Gently toss to combine.
3. In a small bowl, whisk together the olive oil, lemon juice, Dijon, oregano and red pepper flakes (if using). Season with salt and pepper to taste.
4. Pour the dressing over the tuna salad and toss gently until everything is evenly coated.
5. Serve immediately on a bed of greens, in a pita or on top of crackers. Or refrigerate until ready to serve.

Cooking and Prep Time

- Prep Time: 10 minutes
- Total Time: 10 minutes

Serving

This recipe makes about 4 servings as a main dish or 6-8 servings as a side or appetizer.

Nutrition (per serving)

- Calories: 180
- Protein: 20g
- Fat: 10g
- Carbs: 5g
- Fiber: 2g

9.2.6 Chickpea and Vegetable Stir-Fry

Ingredients

- **For the Stir-Fry:**
    - 1 can (15 oz) chickpeas, drained and rinsed
    - 1 cup broccoli florets
    - 1 cup bell peppers (red, yellow, or green), sliced
    - 1 cup carrots, sliced
    - 1 cup snap peas or snow peas
    - 1 medium onion, sliced
    - 3 cloves garlic, minced
    - 1 tablespoon fresh ginger, minced
    - 2 tablespoons olive oil or canola oil
    - Salt and pepper to taste

- **For the Sauce:**
    - 3 tablespoons soy sauce or tamari
    - 1 tablespoon honey or maple syrup
    - 1 tablespoon rice vinegar or lime juice
    - 1 teaspoon sesame oil (optional)
    - 1/4 teaspoon red pepper flakes (optional)

Directions

1. **Prepare the Sauce:** In a small bowl, whisk together the soy sauce, honey, rice vinegar, sesame oil, and red pepper flakes. Set aside.
2. **Cook the Vegetables:** In a large skillet or wok, heat the olive oil over medium-high heat. Add the sliced onion and cook for 2-3 minutes until slightly translucent.

3. **Add Garlic and Ginger:** Stir in the minced garlic and ginger, cooking for another minute until fragrant.
4. **Add Remaining Vegetables:** Add the broccoli, bell peppers, carrots, and snap peas to the skillet. Stir-fry for about 5-7 minutes, or until the vegetables are tender-crisp.
5. **Add Chickpeas and Sauce:** Stir in the chickpeas and the prepared sauce. Cook for an additional 2-3 minutes, stirring frequently, until everything is heated through and well combined.
6. **Serve:** Remove from heat and season with salt and pepper to taste. Serve hot, over rice or quinoa if desired.

Cooking and Prep Time

- **Prep Time:** 10 minutes
- **Cook Time:** 10 minutes
- **Total Time:** 20 minutes

Serving

This recipe serves about 4 people as a main dish or can serve 6 as a side.

Nutrition (per serving)

- **Calories:** Approximately 220
- **Protein:** 10g
- **Fat:** 8g
- **Carbohydrates:** 30g
- **Fiber:** 8g
- **Sugar:** 5g
- **Sodium:** 400mg

9.2.7 Spinach and Strawberry Salad

Ingredients

- **Salad:**
    - 5 oz baby spinach
    - 8 oz strawberries, sliced
    - 1 large avocado, sliced
    - ½ small red onion, thinly sliced
    - ½ cup feta cheese, crumbled
    - ⅓ cup sliced almonds (toasted if desired)
    - ¼ cup pistachios (optional)

- **Dressing:**
    - 3 tbsp balsamic vinegar
    - ¼ cup olive oil
    - 1 garlic clove, minced
    - ½ tsp Dijon mustard
    - ½ tbsp strawberry jam
    - Salt and pepper to taste

Directions

1. **Make the Dressing:** Mix balsamic vinegar, olive oil, garlic, Dijon mustard, strawberry jam, salt, and pepper in a bowl or jar.
2. **Toast Almonds:** If using raw almonds, toast them in a skillet over medium heat for 2-5 minutes until golden.
3. **Combine Salad Ingredients:** In a large bowl, combine spinach, strawberries, avocado, red onion, feta, almonds, and pistachios.
4. **Add Dressing:** Pour the dressing over the salad and toss gently.
5. **Serve:** Enjoy immediately or chill for up to 30 minutes before serving.

Cooking and Prep Time

- **Prep Time:** 15 minutes
- **Total Time:** 15 minutes

Serving

Serves about 4 as a main dish or 6 as a side salad.

Nutrition (per serving)

- **Calories:** ~250
- **Protein:** 6g
- **Fat:** 18g
- **Carbohydrates:** 20g
- **Fiber:** 5g

9.2.8 Grilled Veggie Sandwich

Ingredients

- **For the Hummus:**
    - 1 ½ cups canned chickpeas, drained and rinsed
    - 2 tablespoons olive oil
    - 2 teaspoons tahini
    - Juice from ½ lemon
    - Salt to taste

- **For the Grilled Vegetables:**
    - 2 tablespoons olive oil
    - 1 teaspoon ground cumin
    - ½ teaspoon ground coriander
    - ¼ teaspoon salt
    - 1 zucchini, sliced
    - 1 red bell pepper, cut into strips
    - 1 yellow onion, cut into rounds
    - 1 yellow squash, sliced
    - 8 slices of bread (ciabatta or your choice), toasted

Directions

1. **Make Hummus:** Blend chickpeas, olive oil, tahini, lemon juice, and salt until smooth. Set aside.
2. **Prepare Veggies:** In a bowl, mix olive oil, cumin, coriander, and salt. Toss zucchini, bell pepper, onion, and yellow squash in the mix.
3. **Grill Veggies:** Preheat grill or grill pan. Grill vegetables for 2-3 minutes on each side until tender.

4. **Assemble Sandwich:** Spread hummus on toasted bread. Add grilled vegetables and top with another slice of bread.
5. **Serve:** Cut sandwiches in half and enjoy warm.

Cooking and Prep Time

- **Prep Time:** 10 minutes
- **Cook Time:** 15 minutes
- **Total Time:** 25 minutes

Serving

Makes about 4 sandwiches.

Nutrition (per sandwich)

- **Calories:** Approximately 250
- **Protein:** 10g
- **Fat:** 8g
- **Carbohydrates:** 35g
- **Fiber:** 6g

9.2.9 Greek Salad with Tzatziki Dressing

Ingredients

For the Salad:

- 3 cups baby leaf lettuce
- 1/2 pint cherry tomatoes, halved
- 1 cup black olives, pitted
- 1 cup feta cheese, cubed
- 1/2 red onion, halved and thinly sliced
- 1 cup cucumber, diced

For the Tzatziki Dressing:

- 2 cups Greek yogurt
- 1 large cucumber, peeled, seeded, and grated
- 3 cloves garlic, crushed
- Juice of 1 lemon
- 2 tablespoons fresh dill, chopped
- 1 teaspoon sea salt
- 2 tablespoons olive oil

Directions

1. **Drain Cucumber:** Place the grated cucumber in a colander and let it drain for about 30 minutes to remove excess moisture.
2. **Make Tzatziki Dressing:** In a bowl, combine Greek yogurt, drained cucumber, garlic, lemon juice, dill, salt, and olive oil. Mix well.
3. **Prepare Salad:** In a large bowl, combine the lettuce, cherry tomatoes, black olives, feta cheese, red onion, and diced cucumber.
4. **Serve:** Toss the salad ingredients together. Serve with tzatziki dressing on the side or drizzled over the salad.

Cooking and Prep Time

- **Prep Time:** 15 minutes
- **Total Time:** 15 minutes

Serving

This recipe serves about 4 people.

Nutrition (per serving)

- **Calories:** Approximately 322
- **Protein:** 19g
- **Fat:** 21g
- **Carbohydrates:** 17g
- **Fiber:** 5g
- **Sugar:** 9g

9.2.10 Baked Sweet Potato with Black Beans

Ingredients

- 4 medium sweet potatoes
- 1 (15 oz) can black beans, drained and rinsed
- 1/2 cup salsa
- 1/2 cup shredded cheddar cheese
- 2 tablespoons chopped fresh cilantro (optional)
- Salt and pepper to taste

Directions

1. **Preheat the oven** to 400°F (200°C).
2. **Pierce the sweet potatoes** several times with a fork. Place them directly on the oven rack and bake for 45-60 minutes, or until tender when pierced with a fork.
3. **Remove the sweet potatoes** from the oven and let them cool for a few minutes.
4. **Cut each sweet potato** in half lengthwise. Use a fork to mash the insides slightly.
5. **Top each sweet potato half** with black beans, salsa, shredded cheese, and cilantro (if using). Season with salt and pepper to taste.
6. **Return the stuffed sweet potatoes** to the oven and bake for an additional 5-10 minutes, or until the cheese is melted and bubbly.
7. **Serve hot and enjoy!**

Cooking and Prep Time

- **Prep Time:** 10 minutes
- **Cook Time:** 50-70 minutes
- **Total Time:** 60-80 minutes

Serving

This recipe makes 4 servings, with each serving consisting of half a sweet potato.

Nutrition (per serving)

- **Calories:** Approximately 260
- **Protein:** 10g
- **Fat:** 4g
- **Carbohydrates:** 45g
- **Fiber:** 8g

9.2.11 Zucchini Noodles with Pesto

Ingredients

- 3-4 medium zucchinis, ends trimmed
- 2 cups packed fresh basil leaves
- 2 cloves garlic
- 1/3 cup extra-virgin olive oil
- 2 tbsp freshly grated Parmesan cheese
- 1-2 tsp lemon juice
- Salt and pepper to taste
- Cherry tomatoes (optional)

Instructions

1. **Use a spiralizer, julienne peeler or mandoline** to slice the zucchini into noodles. Set aside.
2. **In a food processor**, combine the basil and garlic. Pulse until coarsely chopped. Slowly add the olive oil while processing. Stop and scrape down the sides. Add the Parmesan, lemon juice, salt and pepper. Pulse until blended.
3. **In a skillet over medium heat**, sauté the zucchini noodles for 1-2 minutes until just softened, being careful not to overcook. Alternatively, you can enjoy them raw.
4. **Toss the zucchini noodles with the pesto** until well coated. Top with cherry tomatoes if desired. Serve immediately.

Prep Time: 10 minutes

Cook Time: 2 minutes

Total Time: 12 minutes

Servings: 4

Nutrition (per serving)

- Calories: 224

- Carbs: 7g
- Protein: 5g
- Fat: 20g
- Saturated Fat: 3g
- Cholesterol: 5mg
- Sodium: 159mg

9.2.12 Low-Sodium Minestrone Soup

Ingredients

- 1 cup diced celery
- 1 cup diced carrots
- 1 cup diced onion
- 1 cup cut green beans (1-inch pieces)
- 8 cups no-salt-added chicken or vegetable stock
- 2 (14.5 oz) cans no-salt-added diced tomatoes
- 1 (15 oz) can no-salt-added kidney beans, rinsed and drained
- 1 (15 oz) can no-salt-added pinto beans, rinsed and drained
- 4 cloves minced garlic
- 1 tbsp dried basil
- 2 tsp dried oregano
- 2 tsp dried thyme
- 1/2 tsp dried rosemary
- 1 tsp black pepper
- 2 cups uncooked small pasta like ditalini, elbow or shells

Instructions

1. Add all ingredients except pasta to a slow cooker. Cook on low for 8-10 hours or high for 4-5 hours, stirring occasionally.
2. About 10-15 minutes before serving, stir in the uncooked pasta. Cook on high until pasta is al dente.
3. Ladle into bowls and serve immediately. Top with freshly grated Parmesan cheese if desired.

Prep Time: 10 minutes

Cook Time: 8-10 hours (low), 4-5 hours (high)

Total Time: 8-10 hours 10 minutes

Servings: 10

Nutrition (per serving)

- Calories: 148
- Total Fat: 1g
- Saturated Fat: 0g
- Cholesterol: 11mg
- Sodium: 86mg
- Carbohydrates: 26g
- Fiber: 7g
- Sugar: 6g
- Protein: 10g

9.2.13 Egg Salad Lettuce Wraps

Ingredients

- 6 hard-boiled eggs, peeled and chopped
- 1/4 cup mayonnaise
- 1 tablespoon Dijon mustard (or yellow mustard)
- 1 tablespoon finely chopped dill pickles (optional)
- 1 tablespoon finely chopped green onions (optional)
- Salt and pepper to taste
- 4-6 large lettuce leaves (such as romaine or butter lettuce)

Instructions

1. **Prepare the Eggs:** In a medium bowl, mash the hard-boiled eggs with a fork until they are crumbly.
2. **Mix the Dressing:** Add the mayonnaise, mustard, dill pickles, green onions, salt, and pepper to the mashed eggs. Mix until well combined and creamy.
3. **Assemble the Wraps:** Take a lettuce leaf and spoon a generous amount of the egg salad mixture onto the center.
4. **Wrap and Serve:** Fold the sides of the lettuce leaf over the filling and enjoy as a wrap. Repeat with remaining leaves and egg salad.

Prep Time: 10 minutes

Cook Time: 10 minutes (for boiling eggs)

Total Time: 20 minutes

Servings: 2-3

Nutrition (per serving, assuming 3 servings total)

- Calories: 240
- Total Fat: 20g
- Saturated Fat: 3g
- Cholesterol: 370mg

- Sodium: 400mg
- Carbohydrates: 2g
- Fiber: 0g
- Sugar: 1g
- Protein: 11g

9.2.14 Cauliflower Rice Bowl

Ingredients

- 4 cups cauliflower rice (about 1 small head of cauliflower)
- 2 tbsp olive oil, divided
- 1 tsp ground cumin
- 1/2 tsp chili powder
- 1/4 tsp turmeric
- Salt and pepper to taste
- 1 cup cooked black beans or pinto beans
- 1 cup diced bell peppers (any color)
- 1/2 cup diced red onion
- 1 avocado, diced
- 1/4 cup chopped fresh cilantro
- Lime wedges for serving

Instructions

1. **Make the cauliflower rice**: Grate or pulse cauliflower florets in a food processor until they resemble rice-sized pieces.
2. **Cook the cauliflower rice**: In a large skillet, heat 1 tbsp olive oil over medium heat. Add the cauliflower rice, cumin, chili powder, turmeric, salt and pepper. Cook for 3-4 minutes, stirring frequently, until tender-crisp. Transfer to a bowl.
3. **Sauté the peppers and onions**: In the same skillet, heat the remaining 1 tbsp olive oil over medium-high heat. Add the bell peppers and onion. Cook for 4-5 minutes until slightly softened and charred in spots.
4. **Assemble the bowls**: Divide the cauliflower rice between 4 bowls. Top each with black beans, sautéed peppers and onions, avocado, and cilantro.
5. **Serve with lime wedges** for squeezing over the top.

Prep Time: 10 minutes

Cook Time: 10 minutes

Total Time: 20 minutes

Servings: 4

Nutrition (per serving)

- Calories: 250
- Carbs: 25g
- Protein: 8g
- Fat: 15g
- Fiber: 10g
- Sodium: 300mg

9.2.15 Hummus and Veggie Wrap

Ingredients

- 1 large tortilla (12-inch)
- 1/2 cup hummus (any flavor)
- 1/8 cup cucumber, sliced
- 1/8 cup diced tomato
- 1/8 cup bell pepper, sliced
- 1/8 cup shoestring carrots
- 3 slices red onion
- Alfalfa sprouts (optional)
- Lettuce leaves (optional)

Instructions

1. **Prepare the Tortilla**: If desired, microwave the tortilla for a few seconds to make it more pliable.
2. **Spread the Hummus**: Evenly spread the hummus over the tortilla, leaving about an inch around the edges.
3. **Add the Veggies**: Layer the cucumber, diced tomato, bell pepper, shoestring carrots, red onion, and any additional toppings like alfalfa sprouts or lettuce on top of the hummus.
4. **Wrap It Up**: Starting from one end, roll the tortilla tightly around the filling. Slice the wrap in half or enjoy it whole.

Prep Time: 5 minutes

Cook Time: 0 minutes

Total Time: 5 minutes

Servings: 1

Nutrition (per serving)

- Calories: 309

- Carbohydrates: 32g
- Protein: 10g
- Fat: 17g
- Saturated Fat: 3g
- Sodium: 520mg
- Potassium: 477mg
- Fiber: 9g
- Sugar: 2g

Dinner Recipes

10.2.1 Herb-Roasted Chicken

Ingredients

- 1 whole chicken (5-6 pounds)
- 1/2 yellow onion, cut into wedges
- 4 cloves garlic, crushed
- 1 handful fresh herbs (thyme, rosemary, or parsley)
- 1.5 tablespoons olive oil
- 1 teaspoon kosher salt
- 1/2 teaspoon freshly ground black pepper
- 1 teaspoon garlic powder
- 1/2 teaspoon paprika

Directions

1. **Preheat the Oven**: Preheat your oven to 425°F (220°C). Arrange the oven rack in the bottom third of the oven.
2. **Prepare the Chicken**: Remove the giblets from the chicken cavity and rinse the chicken under cold water. Pat it dry with paper towels.
3. **Stuff the Cavity**: Place the onion wedges, crushed garlic, and fresh herbs into the cavity of the chicken.
4. **Season the Chicken**: Rub the chicken all over with olive oil. In a small bowl, combine the salt, pepper, garlic powder, and paprika. Season the chicken generously with this mixture, ensuring to coat it evenly.
5. **Roast the Chicken**: Place the chicken breast side up on a rack in a roasting pan. Roast in the preheated oven for 1.5 to 2 hours, or until the internal temperature reaches 180°F (82°C) in the thickest part of the thigh. If the chicken browns too quickly, loosely cover it with aluminum foil.

6. **Rest and Serve**: Once cooked, remove the chicken from the oven and cover it with aluminum foil. Let it rest for at least 10 minutes before carving.

Prep Time: 15 minutes

Cook Time: 1.5 to 2 hours

Total Time: 1 hour 45 minutes to 2 hours 15 minutes

Servings: 6-8

Nutrition (per serving, based on 8 servings)

- Calories: 350
- Protein: 30g
- Total Fat: 22g
- Saturated Fat: 5g
- Cholesterol: 120mg
- Sodium: 450mg
- Carbohydrates: 1g
- Fiber: 0g
- Sugar: 0g

10.2.2 Baked Salmon with Dill

Ingredients

- 4 (6-ounce) salmon fillets
- 2 tbsp unsalted butter, melted
- 1 tbsp lemon juice (about 1/2 lemon)
- 2 tsp chopped fresh dill, plus more for garnish
- 1 tsp grated lemon zest
- 1/4 tsp salt
- 1/8 tsp black pepper

Instructions

1. **Preheat oven** to 400°F. Line a baking sheet with parchment paper.
2. **In a small bowl**, whisk together the melted butter, lemon juice, 2 tsp dill, lemon zest, salt and pepper.
3. **Place the salmon fillets** skin-side down on the prepared baking sheet. Brush the tops and sides of the salmon with the dill butter sauce.
4. **Bake for 12-15 minutes**, until the salmon is opaque and flakes easily with a fork. The internal temperature should reach 145°F.
5. **Garnish with additional fresh dill** before serving.

Prep Time: 5 minutes

Cook Time: 12-15 minutes

Total Time: 20 minutes

Servings: 4

Nutrition (per serving)

- Calories: 290
- Total Fat: 18g
- Saturated Fat: 6g
- Cholesterol: 90mg

- Sodium: 300mg
- Carbohydrates: 1g
- Fiber: 0g
- Protein: 30g

10.2.3 Veggie-Stuffed Bell Peppers

Ingredients

- 6 bell peppers (any color)
- 1 cup cooked brown rice
- 1 (15 oz) can black beans, rinsed and drained
- 1 cup diced zucchini
- 1/2 cup diced onion
- 1/2 cup diced tomatoes
- 2 cloves garlic, minced
- 1 tsp ground cumin
- 1 tsp dried oregano
- 1/4 tsp red pepper flakes (optional)
- Salt and pepper to taste
- 1/2 cup shredded cheddar cheese (optional)

Instructions

1. **Preheat oven** to 375°F. Cut the tops off the bell peppers and remove seeds and membranes. Place peppers in a baking dish and set aside.
2. **In a large bowl**, combine the cooked rice, black beans, zucchini, onion, tomatoes, garlic, cumin, oregano, red pepper flakes (if using), salt and pepper. Mix well.
3. **Stuff each bell pepper** cavity with the vegetable mixture, packing it in tightly. Top with shredded cheese if desired.
4. **Pour a small amount of water** into the bottom of the baking dish. Cover with foil.
5. **Bake for 30 minutes**, then remove foil and bake for an additional 10-15 minutes until peppers are tender.
6. **Serve hot** and enjoy!

Prep Time: 15 minutes

Cook Time: 45 minutes

Total Time: 1 hour

Servings: 6

Nutrition (per serving)

- Calories: 190
- Total Fat: 3g
- Saturated Fat: 1g
- Cholesterol: 5mg
- Sodium: 360mg
- Carbohydrates: 35g
- Fiber: 8g
- Sugar: 6g
- Protein: 9g

10.2.4 Garlic and Herb Pork Tenderloin

Ingredients

- 2 lbs pork tenderloin
- ¼ cup Dijon mustard
- 2 tsp garlic, minced
- 1 tsp dried thyme
- 1 tsp dried rosemary
- ½ tsp salt
- ¼ tsp black pepper
- 1 tbsp olive oil
- ⅓ cup Parmesan cheese, shredded (optional)

Directions

1. **Preheat the Oven**: Preheat your oven to 425°F (220°C).
2. **Prepare the Pork**: Pat the pork tenderloins dry with paper towels. Slather the pork with Dijon mustard, coating it completely.
3. **Season the Pork**: In a small bowl, mix together the minced garlic, thyme, rosemary, salt, and pepper. Rub this mixture all over the pork tenderloins.
4. **Sear the Pork**: Heat olive oil in a large cast-iron skillet or oven-safe pan over medium-high heat. Sear the pork tenderloins on all sides until nicely browned (about 3-4 minutes per side).
5. **Bake the Pork**: Sprinkle the tops of the tenderloins with shredded Parmesan cheese, if using. Transfer the skillet to the preheated oven and bake for 10-15 minutes, or until the internal temperature reaches 140°F (60°C).
6. **Rest and Serve**: Remove the pork from the oven and cover it loosely with foil. Let it rest for 5-10 minutes before slicing into medallions. Serve warm.

Prep Time: 10 minutes

Cook Time: 25 minutes

Total Time: 35 minutes

Servings: 4-6

Nutrition (per serving, based on 6 servings)

- Calories: 290
- Protein: 30g
- Total Fat: 18g
- Saturated Fat: 6g
- Cholesterol: 90mg
- Sodium: 450mg
- Carbohydrates: 1g
- Fiber: 0g
- Sugar: 0g

10.2.5 Spaghetti Squash with Marinara

Ingredients

- 1 medium spaghetti squash
- 2 cups marinara sauce (store-bought or homemade)
- 1 tablespoon olive oil
- 2 cloves garlic, minced
- 1/4 teaspoon red pepper flakes (optional)
- Salt and pepper to taste
- Fresh basil or parsley for garnish (optional)
- Grated Parmesan cheese for serving (optional)

Directions

1. **Preheat the Oven**: Preheat your oven to 400°F (200°C).
2. **Prepare the Spaghetti Squash**: Cut the spaghetti squash in half lengthwise and scoop out the seeds. Drizzle the inside with olive oil and season with salt and pepper.
3. **Roast the Squash**: Place the squash halves cut-side down on a baking sheet lined with parchment paper. Roast in the preheated oven for 30-40 minutes, or until the flesh is tender and easily shreds with a fork.
4. **Heat the Marinara Sauce**: While the squash is roasting, heat the marinara sauce in a saucepan over medium heat. Add minced garlic and red pepper flakes, and simmer for about 5-10 minutes until heated through. Adjust seasoning with salt and pepper.
5. **Shred the Squash**: Once the spaghetti squash is cooked, remove it from the oven and let it cool slightly. Using a fork, scrape the flesh to create spaghetti-like strands.
6. **Combine and Serve**: In a large bowl, toss the spaghetti squash strands with the marinara sauce. Serve hot, garnished with fresh basil or parsley and grated Parmesan cheese if desired.

Prep Time: 10 minutes

Cook Time: 30-40 minutes

Total Time: 40-50 minutes

Servings: 4

Nutrition (per serving)

- Calories: 150
- Total Fat: 7g
- Saturated Fat: 1g
- Cholesterol: 5mg
- Sodium: 300mg
- Carbohydrates: 20g
- Fiber: 5g
- Sugar: 6g
- Protein: 4g

10.2.6 Grilled Shrimp Skewers

Ingredients

- 1 lb large shrimp, peeled and deveined
- 1/4 cup olive oil
- 2 tbsp lemon juice
- 3 cloves garlic, minced
- 1 tsp paprika
- 1/2 tsp dried oregano
- 1/4 tsp red pepper flakes (optional)
- Salt and pepper to taste
- Lemon wedges for serving

Instructions

1. **In a large bowl,** whisk together the olive oil, lemon juice, garlic, paprika, oregano, red pepper flakes (if using), salt and pepper.
2. **Add the shrimp** and toss to coat evenly. Cover and refrigerate for 15-30 minutes.
3. **If using wooden skewers**, soak them in water for at least 30 minutes to prevent burning.
4. **Thread the marinated shrimp** onto the skewers, leaving a small space between each one.
5. **Preheat grill** to medium-high heat. Lightly oil the grates.
6. **Grill the shrimp skewers** for 2-3 minutes per side, until they turn pink and opaque. Be careful not to overcook.
7. **Serve immediately** with lemon wedges for squeezing over the top.

Prep Time: 10 minutes

Marinating Time: 15-30 minutes

Cook Time: 6-8 minutes

Total Time: 30-45 minutes

Servings: 4

Nutrition (per serving)

- Calories: 220
- Total Fat: 12g
- Saturated Fat: 2g
- Cholesterol: 286mg
- Sodium: 1173mg
- Carbohydrates: 3g
- Fiber: 0g
- Protein: 24g

10.2.7 Quinoa-Stuffed Acorn Squash

Ingredients

- 2 medium acorn squash (about 2 lbs total)
- 1/2 cup quinoa (uncooked)
- 1 cup vegetable broth or water
- 2 tablespoons olive oil
- 1 medium onion, diced
- 2 cloves garlic, minced
- 1/2 teaspoon ground cumin
- 1/4 teaspoon ground cinnamon
- 1/8 teaspoon ground ginger
- 1/3 cup dried apricots, chopped (or cranberries)
- 1/3 cup natural almonds, chopped (or pecans)
- 1 tablespoon fresh lemon juice
- 1/4 cup chopped fresh parsley
- 2 tablespoons chopped fresh mint (optional)
- Salt and pepper to taste
- Honey for drizzling (optional)

Directions

1. **Preheat the Oven**: Preheat your oven to 375°F (190°C).
2. **Prepare the Squash**: Cut the acorn squash in half lengthwise and scoop out the seeds. Brush the cut sides with 1 tablespoon of olive oil and season with salt and pepper. Place the squash halves cut-side down on a baking sheet and bake for 40 minutes, or until tender.
3. **Cook the Quinoa**: While the squash is baking, rinse the quinoa under cold water. In a medium saucepan, combine the quinoa and vegetable broth. Bring to a boil, then reduce the heat to low, cover, and simmer for about 15 minutes, or until all the liquid is absorbed. Fluff with a fork and set aside.

4. **Sauté the Vegetables**: In a skillet, heat the remaining tablespoon of olive oil over medium heat. Add the diced onion and sauté until softened, about 3 minutes. Add the minced garlic and cook for an additional 30 seconds. Stir in the cumin, cinnamon, and ginger, and remove from heat.
5. **Combine the Filling**: In a large bowl, combine the cooked quinoa, sautéed onion mixture, chopped apricots, almonds, lemon juice, parsley, and mint (if using). Season with salt and pepper to taste.
6. **Stuff the Squash**: Remove the squash from the oven and carefully turn them cut-side up. Fill each half with the quinoa mixture, packing it in gently. Drizzle with honey if desired.
7. **Bake Again**: Return the stuffed squash to the oven and bake for an additional 10-15 minutes, until heated through.
8. **Serve**: Garnish with additional fresh herbs if desired and serve warm.

Prep Time: 15 minutes

Cook Time: 55 minutes

Total Time: 1 hour 10 minutes

Servings: 4

Nutrition (per serving)

- Calories: 320
- Total Fat: 12g
- Saturated Fat: 1g
- Cholesterol: 0mg
- Sodium: 150mg
- Carbohydrates: 48g
- Fiber: 8g
- Sugar: 10g
- Protein: 8g

10.2.8 Lemon Herb Tilapia

Ingredients

- 4 tilapia fillets (about 1 lb total)
- 2 tbsp olive oil
- 2 tbsp lemon juice
- 1 tsp Dijon mustard
- 1 tsp Italian seasoning
- 1 tsp lemon zest
- 1 tsp garlic powder
- 1 tsp onion powder
- 1/2 tsp salt
- 1/4 tsp black pepper
- 2 tbsp chopped fresh dill, parsley or chives for garnish
- Lemon wedges for serving

Instructions

1. **In a shallow dish**, whisk together the olive oil, lemon juice, mustard, Italian seasoning, lemon zest, garlic powder, onion powder, salt and pepper.
2. **Add the tilapia fillets** and turn to coat both sides with the marinade. Cover and refrigerate for 15-30 minutes.
3. **Preheat oven** to 400°F. Line a baking sheet with parchment paper.
4. **Place the marinated tilapia** on the prepared baking sheet. Bake for 12-15 minutes, until fish flakes easily with a fork.
5. **Transfer to a serving platter**, drizzle with any remaining marinade from the baking sheet.
6. **Garnish with chopped fresh herbs** and serve immediately with lemon wedges.

Prep Time: 10 minutes

Marinating Time: 15-30 minutes

Cook Time: 12-15 minutes

Total Time: 40 minutes

Servings: 4

Nutrition (per serving)

- Calories: 190
- Total Fat: 8g
- Saturated Fat: 1g
- Cholesterol: 80mg
- Sodium: 400mg
- Carbohydrates: 2g
- Fiber: 0g
- Protein: 28g

10.2.9 Chicken and Broccoli Stir-Fry

Ingredients

For the Stir-Fry:

- 1 lb boneless, skinless chicken breast, cut into bite-sized pieces
- 2 tablespoons vegetable oil (divided)
- 2 cups broccoli florets
- 1 small onion, sliced
- 1/2 lb mushrooms, sliced (optional)
- Salt and pepper to taste

For the Stir-Fry Sauce:

- 2/3 cup low-sodium chicken broth
- 3 tablespoons low-sodium soy sauce
- 2 tablespoons honey (or brown sugar)
- 1 tablespoon cornstarch
- 1 tablespoon sesame oil
- 1 teaspoon fresh ginger, minced
- 2 cloves garlic, minced
- 1/4 teaspoon black pepper

Directions

1. **Prepare the Sauce**: In a small bowl, whisk together the chicken broth, soy sauce, honey, cornstarch, sesame oil, ginger, garlic, and black pepper. Set aside.
2. **Cook the Chicken**: Heat 1 tablespoon of vegetable oil in a large skillet or wok over medium-high heat. Add the chicken pieces and season with salt and pepper. Cook for about 5-7 minutes, stirring occasionally, until the chicken is golden brown and cooked through. Remove the chicken from the skillet and set aside.

3. **Sauté the Vegetables**: In the same skillet, add the remaining tablespoon of oil. Add the broccoli, onion, and mushrooms (if using). Stir-fry for 3-4 minutes, or until the vegetables are tender-crisp.
4. **Combine Chicken and Sauce**: Return the cooked chicken to the skillet with the vegetables. Pour the stir-fry sauce over the mixture and stir well to combine. Cook for an additional 2-3 minutes, or until the sauce has thickened and everything is heated through.
5. **Serve**: Serve the chicken and broccoli stir-fry over cooked rice or noodles, garnished with sesame seeds or green onions if desired.

Prep Time: 10 minutes

Cook Time: 15 minutes

Total Time: 25 minutes

Servings: 4

Nutrition (per serving)

- Calories: 280
- Total Fat: 10g
- Saturated Fat: 1.5g
- Cholesterol: 70mg
- Sodium: 600mg
- Carbohydrates: 20g
- Fiber: 3g
- Sugar: 6g
- Protein: 25g

10.2.10 Low-Sodium Beef Stew

Ingredients

- 1 lb beef stew meat, cut into 1-inch cubes
- 2 tbsp olive oil
- 1 onion, diced
- 3 cloves garlic, minced
- 2 cups low-sodium beef broth
- 1 cup water
- 2 bay leaves
- 1 tsp dried thyme
- 1/2 tsp black pepper
- 2 medium potatoes, peeled and cubed
- 3 carrots, peeled and sliced
- 2 stalks celery, sliced
- 1 cup frozen peas
- 2 tbsp cornstarch (optional)

Instructions

1. **In a large pot or Dutch oven**, heat the olive oil over medium-high heat. Add the beef in a single layer and cook until browned on all sides, about 2-3 minutes per side. Transfer beef to a plate.
2. **Add the onion** to the pot and cook for 2-3 minutes until translucent. Add the garlic and cook for 1 minute until fragrant.
3. **Pour in the beef broth and water**, scraping up any browned bits from the bottom of the pot. Add the bay leaves, thyme and black pepper.
4. **Return the beef and any juices** to the pot. Bring to a boil, then reduce heat to low, cover and simmer for 1 hour.
5. **Add the potatoes, carrots and celery.** Cover and simmer for 30 minutes, until beef and vegetables are tender.

6. **Stir in the frozen peas** and cook for 5 more minutes.
7. **If desired, make a slurry** with the cornstarch and 2 tbsp water. Slowly whisk it into the stew to thicken the broth.
8. **Taste and adjust seasoning** as needed. Remove bay leaves before serving.

Prep Time: 15 minutes

Cook Time: 1 hour 45 minutes

Total Time: 2 hours

Servings: 6

Nutrition (per serving)

- Calories: 350
- Total Fat: 12g
- Saturated Fat: 3g
- Cholesterol: 70mg
- Sodium: 250mg
- Carbohydrates: 30g
- Fiber: 5g
- Protein: 30g

10.2.11 Veggie and Black Bean Enchiladas

Ingredients

- 8 small corn tortillas
- 1 can (15 oz) black beans, rinsed and drained
- 1 cup corn (fresh, frozen, or canned)
- 1 medium zucchini, diced
- 1 red bell pepper, diced
- 1 small onion, diced
- 2 cloves garlic, minced
- 1 teaspoon cumin
- 1 teaspoon chili powder
- 1/2 teaspoon salt (optional)
- 1 cup enchilada sauce (store-bought or homemade)
- 1 cup shredded cheese (cheddar or Mexican blend)
- Fresh cilantro for garnish (optional)
- Lime wedges for serving (optional)

Directions

1. **Preheat the Oven**: Preheat your oven to 375°F (190°C).
2. **Sauté the Vegetables**: In a large skillet, heat a tablespoon of olive oil over medium heat. Add the onion and garlic, and sauté for 2-3 minutes until the onion is translucent. Add the zucchini and bell pepper, cooking for an additional 5 minutes until softened. Stir in the corn, black beans, cumin, chili powder, and salt. Cook for another 2-3 minutes until heated through. Remove from heat.
3. **Prepare the Tortillas**: In a separate pan, lightly warm the corn tortillas for about 30 seconds on each side to make them pliable.
4. **Assemble the Enchiladas**: Spread a small amount of enchilada sauce on the bottom of a baking dish. Take a tortilla, fill it with a generous amount of the veggie and bean mixture, and sprinkle a little cheese on top. Roll the tortilla

tightly and place it seam-side down in the baking dish. Repeat with the remaining tortillas.

5. **Top with Sauce and Cheese**: Once all the enchiladas are in the baking dish, pour the remaining enchilada sauce over the top and sprinkle with the remaining cheese.
6. **Bake**: Cover the baking dish with foil and bake for 20 minutes. Remove the foil and bake for an additional 10 minutes, or until the cheese is bubbly and golden.
7. **Serve**: Garnish with fresh cilantro and serve with lime wedges on the side.

Prep Time: 15 minutes

Cook Time: 30 minutes

Total Time: 45 minutes

Servings: 4

Nutrition (per serving)

- Calories: 320
- Total Fat: 10g
- Saturated Fat: 4g
- Cholesterol: 20mg
- Sodium: 450mg
- Carbohydrates: 45g
- Fiber: 10g
- Sugar: 4g
- Protein: 12g

10.2.12 Baked Cod with Lemon and Capers

Ingredients

- 4 cod fillets (about 6 ounces each)
- 2 tablespoons olive oil
- 2 tablespoons fresh lemon juice
- 1 tablespoon capers, drained and rinsed
- 2 cloves garlic, minced
- 1 teaspoon dried oregano
- 1/2 teaspoon salt
- 1/4 teaspoon black pepper
- Lemon slices for garnish
- Fresh parsley for garnish (optional)

Directions

1. **Preheat the Oven**: Preheat your oven to 400°F (200°C).
2. **Prepare the Baking Dish**: Lightly grease a baking dish with a little olive oil.
3. **Make the Marinade**: In a small bowl, whisk together the olive oil, lemon juice, capers, minced garlic, oregano, salt, and pepper.
4. **Arrange the Cod**: Place the cod fillets in the prepared baking dish. Pour the marinade over the fillets, ensuring they are well coated.
5. **Bake the Cod**: Bake in the preheated oven for 12-15 minutes, or until the fish flakes easily with a fork and is opaque.
6. **Serve**: Garnish with lemon slices and fresh parsley if desired. Serve immediately with your choice of sides, such as steamed vegetables or rice.

Prep Time: 10 minutes

Cook Time: 15 minutes

Total Time: 25 minutes

Servings: 4

Nutrition (per serving)

- Calories: 220
- Total Fat: 10g
- Saturated Fat: 1.5g
- Cholesterol: 70mg
- Sodium: 290mg
- Carbohydrates: 2g
- Fiber: 0g
- Sugar: 0g
- Protein: 30g

10.2.13 Roasted Turkey Breast

Ingredients

- 6 lb bone-in turkey breast (half breast)
- 5 tablespoons unsalted butter, softened
- 1 teaspoon minced garlic
- 1 tablespoon fresh sage, finely minced
- 1 1/2 teaspoons fresh rosemary, finely minced
- 1 tablespoon fresh thyme, finely minced
- 2 tablespoons fresh parsley, finely minced
- 1 teaspoon kosher salt
- 1/2 teaspoon black pepper
- Cooking spray
- Rosemary sprigs for garnish (optional)

Directions

1. **Preheat the Oven**: Preheat your oven to 450°F (232°C). Coat a baking dish with cooking spray.
2. **Prepare the Herb Butter**: In a bowl, mix together the softened butter, minced garlic, sage, rosemary, thyme, parsley, salt, and pepper until well combined.
3. **Prepare the Turkey**: Loosen the skin of the turkey breast gently with your fingers. Spread half of the herb butter mixture underneath the skin and the other half on top of the turkey breast.
4. **Roast the Turkey**: Place the turkey breast in the prepared baking dish. Roast in the preheated oven for 15-20 minutes, or until the skin starts to brown.
5. **Reduce the Temperature**: Lower the oven temperature to 350°F (175°C) and continue roasting for about 1 hour and 15 minutes, basting occasionally with the pan juices. The internal temperature should reach at least 160°F (71°C) when checked in the thickest part of the meat.

6. **Rest the Turkey**: Once cooked, remove the turkey from the oven and cover it loosely with foil. Let it rest for 5-10 minutes before carving. The internal temperature will rise to 165°F (74°C) during this time.
7. **Serve**: Garnish with rosemary sprigs if desired, and serve warm.

Prep Time: 15 minutes

Cook Time: 1 hour 35 minutes

Total Time: 1 hour 50 minutes

Servings: 6-8

Nutrition (per serving, based on 8 servings)

- Calories: 320
- Total Fat: 20g
- Saturated Fat: 6g
- Cholesterol: 110mg
- Sodium: 400mg
- Carbohydrates: 0g
- Fiber: 0g
- Sugar: 0g
- Protein: 36g

10.2.14 Mushroom and Spinach Risotto

Ingredients

- 1 cup Arborio rice
- 4 cups low-sodium vegetable broth
- 1 cup fresh spinach, chopped
- 1 cup mushrooms, sliced (such as cremini or button)
- 1 small onion, finely chopped
- 2 cloves garlic, minced
- 1/2 cup dry white wine (optional)
- 2 tablespoons olive oil
- 2 tablespoons unsalted butter
- 1/4 cup grated Parmesan cheese (optional)
- Salt and pepper to taste
- Fresh parsley for garnish (optional)

Directions

1. **Heat the Broth**: In a saucepan, bring the vegetable broth to a simmer over low heat. Keep it warm throughout the cooking process.
2. **Sauté the Vegetables**: In a large skillet or saucepan, heat the olive oil and 1 tablespoon of butter over medium heat. Add the chopped onion and cook until translucent, about 3-4 minutes. Add the minced garlic and sliced mushrooms, cooking until the mushrooms are tender and browned, about 5 minutes.
3. **Toast the Rice**: Stir in the Arborio rice and cook for 1-2 minutes, allowing the rice to absorb the flavors and toast slightly.
4. **Add the Wine**: If using, pour in the white wine and stir until it is mostly absorbed by the rice.
5. **Gradually Add Broth**: Begin adding the warm vegetable broth, one ladle at a time, stirring frequently. Allow the liquid to be absorbed before adding the next

ladle. Continue this process for about 18-20 minutes, or until the rice is creamy and al dente.

6. **Stir in Spinach**: Once the rice is cooked, stir in the chopped spinach and the remaining tablespoon of butter. Cook for an additional 2 minutes, until the spinach is wilted.
7. **Finish with Cheese**: Remove from heat and stir in the grated Parmesan cheese, if using. Season with salt and pepper to taste.
8. **Serve**: Garnish with fresh parsley and additional Parmesan cheese if desired. Serve warm.

Prep Time: 10 minutes

Cook Time: 20 minutes

Total Time: 30 minutes

Servings: 4

Nutrition (per serving)

- Calories: 320
- Total Fat: 10g
- Saturated Fat: 4g
- Cholesterol: 15mg
- Sodium: 350mg
- Carbohydrates: 45g
- Fiber: 3g
- Sugar: 2g
- Protein: 10g

10.2.15 Moroccan Chickpea Stew

Ingredients

- 2 tablespoons olive oil
- 1 large onion, diced
- 3 cloves garlic, minced
- 1 tablespoon grated fresh ginger
- 1 teaspoon ground cumin
- 1 teaspoon ground coriander
- 1 teaspoon paprika
- 1/2 teaspoon ground cinnamon
- 1/4 teaspoon cayenne pepper (optional)
- 1 (15 oz) can diced tomatoes
- 1 (15 oz) can chickpeas, rinsed and drained
- 1 cup vegetable broth
- 1 medium sweet potato, peeled and cubed
- 1 cup cauliflower florets
- 1 cup green beans, cut into 1-inch pieces
- 1/4 cup raisins or dried apricots, chopped
- 1/4 cup chopped fresh cilantro
- Salt and pepper to taste
- Lemon wedges for serving

Instructions

1. In a large pot or Dutch oven, heat the olive oil over medium heat. Add the onion and sauté for 5 minutes until translucent.
2. Stir in the garlic, ginger, cumin, coriander, paprika, cinnamon and cayenne (if using). Cook for 1 minute until fragrant.

3. Add the diced tomatoes, chickpeas, vegetable broth, sweet potato, cauliflower and green beans. Bring to a boil, then reduce heat and simmer for 15-20 minutes, until vegetables are tender.
4. Stir in the raisins or apricots and cilantro. Season with salt and pepper to taste.
5. Serve the chickpea stew warm, with lemon wedges on the side for squeezing over top.

Prep Time: 15 minutes

Cook Time: 25 minutes

Total Time: 40 minutes

Servings: 4

Nutrition (per serving)

- Calories: 330
- Total Fat: 8g
- Saturated Fat: 1g
- Cholesterol: 0mg
- Sodium: 600mg
- Carbohydrates: 55g
- Fiber: 12g
- Sugar: 16g
- Protein: 11g

Snack Recipes

11.1.1 Carrot and Cucumber Sticks with Hummus

Ingredients

- 4 large carrots, peeled and cut into sticks
- 2 medium cucumbers, sliced into sticks
- 1 cup hummus (store-bought or homemade)
- Optional: Olive oil, paprika, or sesame seeds for garnish

Directions

1. **Prepare the Vegetables**: Peel the carrots and cut them into sticks about 4-5 inches long. Wash the cucumbers and cut them into sticks of similar length.
2. **Arrange the Veggies**: Place the carrot and cucumber sticks on a serving platter or in a container for easy dipping.
3. **Serve with Hummus**: Place the hummus in a small bowl in the center of the platter or alongside the vegetable sticks.
4. **Optional Garnish**: Drizzle a little olive oil over the hummus and sprinkle with paprika or sesame seeds for added flavor and presentation.

Prep Time: 10 minutes

Total Time: 10 minutes

Servings: 4

Nutrition (per serving)

- Calories: 150
- Total Fat: 7g
- Saturated Fat: 1g
- Cholesterol: 0mg
- Sodium: 200mg

- Carbohydrates: 20g
- Fiber: 5g
- Sugar: 5g
- Protein: 5g

11.1.2 Rice Cakes with Almond Butter

Ingredients

- 2 whole grain rice cakes
- 2 tablespoons creamy almond butter
- 1 banana, sliced (or other fruit like apple, berries, etc.)
- Cinnamon for dusting (optional)

Instructions

1. Spread 1 tablespoon of almond butter evenly on each rice cake.
2. Top with sliced banana or other fruit of your choice.
3. Sprinkle with cinnamon if desired.

Prep Time: 5 minutes

Cook Time: 0 minutes

Total Time: 5 minutes

Servings: 1

Nutrition (per serving)

- Calories: 300
- Total Fat: 14g
- Saturated Fat: 1g
- Cholesterol: 0mg
- Sodium: 0mg
- Carbohydrates: 38g
- Fiber: 6g
- Sugar: 12g
- Protein: 8g

11.1.3 Greek Yogurt with Fresh Berries

Ingredients

- 1 cup plain Greek yogurt
- 1/2 cup fresh berries (such as blueberries, strawberries, or raspberries)
- 1 tablespoon honey (optional)
- 1 tablespoon chopped nuts (such as almonds or walnuts, optional)
- A sprinkle of cinnamon (optional)

Directions

1. **Prepare the Yogurt**: In a bowl, place the Greek yogurt and smooth it out with a spoon.
2. **Add the Berries**: Rinse the fresh berries under cold water. Slice the strawberries if using, and then place the berries on top of the yogurt.
3. **Drizzle with Honey**: If desired, drizzle honey over the top for added sweetness.
4. **Add Nuts and Cinnamon**: Sprinkle chopped nuts and a dash of cinnamon on top if you like.
5. **Serve**: Enjoy immediately as a refreshing snack or breakfast.

Prep Time: 5 minutes

Total Time: 5 minutes

Servings: 1

Nutrition (per serving)

- Calories: 240
- Total Fat: 7g
- Saturated Fat: 1g
- Cholesterol: 10mg
- Sodium: 60mg
- Carbohydrates: 36g
- Fiber: 4g

- Sugar: 25g (includes honey)
- Protein: 16g

11.1.4 Edamame

Ingredients

- 1 lb fresh or frozen edamame in the pod
- 2 tablespoons sea salt (for cooking water)
- 1 tablespoon olive oil or sesame oil (optional)
- 1 teaspoon sea salt or kosher salt (for seasoning cooked edamame)

Instructions

1. **Bring a large pot of water** to a boil and add 2 tablespoons of sea salt.
2. **If using fresh edamame**, remove the stems. For frozen edamame, no preparation is needed.
3. **Add the edamame pods** to the boiling salted water. Cook for 5-7 minutes, or until the beans are tender but still bright green.
4. **Drain the edamame** in a colander and rinse with cold water to stop the cooking process. Pat dry with paper towels.
5. **Transfer the edamame pods** to a serving bowl. Drizzle with olive oil or sesame oil if desired, and sprinkle with 1 teaspoon of salt. Toss to coat evenly.
6. **Serve warm or at room temperature**, providing small dishes for the empty pods. Encourage guests to squeeze the beans directly into their mouths.

Prep Time: 5 minutes

Cook Time: 5-7 minutes

Total Time: 10-12 minutes

Servings: 4

Nutrition (per serving)

- Calories: 189
- Total Fat: 8g
- Saturated Fat: 1g
- Cholesterol: 0mg

- Sodium: 1,500mg
- Carbohydrates: 12g
- Fiber: 5g
- Sugar: 2g
- Protein: 17g

11.1.5 Celery Sticks with Peanut Butter

Ingredients

- 4 large celery stalks
- 1 cup peanut butter (creamy or crunchy, based on preference)
- Optional toppings: raisins, chocolate chips, or granola for added flavor and texture

Directions

1. **Prepare the Celery**: Wash the celery stalks thoroughly under cold water. Trim off the ends and any leaves, then cut each stalk into 3-4 inch pieces.
2. **Spread the Peanut Butter**: Using a knife or spoon, spread about 1-2 tablespoons of peanut butter into the groove of each celery stick, filling it generously.
3. **Add Toppings (Optional)**: If desired, sprinkle raisins, chocolate chips, or granola on top of the peanut butter for added sweetness and crunch.
4. **Serve**: Arrange the celery sticks on a plate and enjoy immediately, or pack them for a snack on the go.

Prep Time: 5 minutes

Total Time: 5 minutes

Servings: 4

Nutrition (per serving)

- Calories: 215
- Total Fat: 16g
- Saturated Fat: 3g
- Cholesterol: 0mg
- Sodium: 166mg
- Carbohydrates: 13g
- Fiber: 3g

- Sugar: 3g
- Protein: 8g

11.1.6 Low-Sodium Popcorn

Ingredients

- 1/2 cup popcorn kernels
- 1 tablespoon vegetable oil (or coconut oil)
- 1 teaspoon garlic powder (optional)
- 1 teaspoon onion powder (optional)
- 1 teaspoon nutritional yeast (optional)
- 1/4 teaspoon paprika (optional)
- Freshly ground black pepper (to taste)

Directions

1. **Heat the Oil**: In a large pot, heat the vegetable oil over medium heat.
2. **Add the Kernels**: Once the oil is hot, add the popcorn kernels to the pot. Cover with a lid, leaving it slightly ajar to allow steam to escape.
3. **Pop the Corn**: Shake the pot occasionally to ensure even popping. The popcorn is done when the popping slows down to about 2 seconds between pops (approximately 3-5 minutes).
4. **Season the Popcorn**: Remove the pot from heat and carefully pour the popcorn into a large bowl. Sprinkle with garlic powder, onion powder, nutritional yeast, paprika, and black pepper, if desired. Toss to coat evenly.
5. **Serve**: Enjoy the popcorn warm as a healthy snack!

Prep Time: 5 minutes

Cook Time: 5 minutes

Total Time: 10 minutes

Servings: 4

Nutrition (per serving)

- Calories: 120
- Total Fat: 6g

- Saturated Fat: 1g
- Cholesterol: 0mg
- Sodium: 0mg
- Carbohydrates: 15g
- Fiber: 3g
- Sugar: 0g
- Protein: 3g

11.1.7 Apple Slices with Cinnamon

Ingredients

- 2 medium apples (any variety, such as Fuji, Honeycrisp, or Granny Smith)
- 1 teaspoon ground cinnamon
- 1 tablespoon honey or maple syrup (optional)
- Lemon juice (optional, to prevent browning)

Directions

1. **Prepare the Apples**: Wash the apples thoroughly. Core and slice them into thin wedges or rounds. If desired, you can sprinkle a little lemon juice on the slices to prevent browning.
2. **Sprinkle with Cinnamon**: Place the apple slices in a bowl and sprinkle the ground cinnamon evenly over them. If you like, drizzle honey or maple syrup for added sweetness.
3. **Toss to Coat**: Gently toss the apple slices to ensure they are evenly coated with cinnamon and sweetener.
4. **Serve**: Enjoy the apple slices immediately, or let them sit for a few minutes to allow the flavors to meld.

Prep Time: 5 minutes

Total Time: 5 minutes

Servings: 2

Nutrition (per serving)

- Calories: 95
- Total Fat: 0g
- Saturated Fat: 0g
- Cholesterol: 0mg
- Sodium: 1mg
- Carbohydrates: 25g

- Fiber: 4g
- Sugar: 19g
- Protein: 0g

11.1.8 Cottage Cheese with Pineapple

Ingredients

- 1 cup low-fat or non-fat cottage cheese
- 1/2 cup fresh pineapple chunks
- 1 teaspoon honey (optional)
- Mint leaves for garnish (optional)

Directions

1. In a small bowl, place the cottage cheese.
2. Top with fresh pineapple chunks.
3. If desired, drizzle with honey for extra sweetness.
4. Garnish with fresh mint leaves (optional).

Prep Time: 5 minutes

Total Time: 5 minutes

Servings: 1

Nutrition (per serving)

- Calories: 210
- Total Fat: 2g
- Saturated Fat: 1g
- Cholesterol: 10mg
- Sodium: 360mg
- Carbohydrates: 24g
- Fiber: 2g
- Sugar: 19g
- Protein: 24g

11.1.9 Mixed Nuts and Seeds

Ingredients

- 1/2 cup almonds (raw or roasted)
- 1/2 cup walnuts (raw or roasted)
- 1/2 cup cashews (raw or roasted)
- 1/2 cup pumpkin seeds (pepitas)
- 1/2 cup sunflower seeds
- 1/4 cup dried cranberries or raisins (optional)
- 1 teaspoon sea salt (optional)
- 1 teaspoon cinnamon (optional)

Directions

1. **Combine Ingredients**: In a large mixing bowl, combine the almonds, walnuts, cashews, pumpkin seeds, and sunflower seeds. If using, add the dried cranberries or raisins for a touch of sweetness.
2. **Season (Optional)**: If you prefer a salted or spiced mix, sprinkle in the sea salt and cinnamon, and stir to combine evenly.
3. **Store**: Transfer the mixed nuts and seeds to an airtight container or resealable bag. Store in a cool, dry place or in the refrigerator for longer freshness.
4. **Serve**: Enjoy as a snack on its own, or use as a topping for salads, yogurt, or oatmeal.

Prep Time: 10 minutes

Total Time: 10 minutes

Servings: 8 (1/4 cup per serving)

Nutrition (per serving)

- Calories: 200
- Total Fat: 16g
- Saturated Fat: 2g

- Cholesterol: 0mg
- Sodium: 50mg (if salted)
- Carbohydrates: 10g
- Fiber: 3g
- Sugar: 2g
- Protein: 6g

11.1.10 Homemade Trail Mix

Ingredients

- 1 cup raw almonds
- 1 cup raw cashews
- 1 cup raw pumpkin seeds (pepitas)
- 1 cup raw sunflower seeds
- 1 cup dried cranberries
- 1 cup dark chocolate chips or cacao nibs
- 1/2 cup unsweetened shredded coconut
- 1/2 cup roasted chickpeas (optional)
- 1/4 cup chia seeds (optional)
- 1/4 cup hemp hearts (optional)

Instructions

1. **In a large bowl**, combine all the ingredients and stir to mix well.
2. **Transfer the trail mix** to an airtight container or resealable bag.
3. **Store in a cool, dry place** for up to 2 weeks.

Prep Time: 10 minutes

Total Time: 10 minutes

Servings: 10 (1/2 cup each)

Nutrition (per serving)

- Calories: 300
- Total Fat: 20g
- Saturated Fat: 5g
- Cholesterol: 0mg
- Sodium: 50mg
- Carbohydrates: 25g
- Fiber: 5g

- Sugar: 10g
- Protein: 10g

11.1.11 Bell Pepper Strips with Guacamole

Ingredients

- 2 large bell peppers (any color: red, yellow, or green)
- 1 cup guacamole (store-bought or homemade)
- Optional: lime wedges for serving
- Optional: chili powder or paprika for seasoning

Directions

1. **Prepare the Bell Peppers**: Wash the bell peppers thoroughly. Cut each pepper in half, remove the seeds and stem, and slice them into strips.
2. **Serve the Guacamole**: In a serving bowl, place the guacamole. If desired, squeeze a little lime juice over the top for added flavor.
3. **Arrange the Veggies**: Place the bell pepper strips around the guacamole on a serving platter.
4. **Optional Seasoning**: If desired, sprinkle a little chili powder or paprika over the guacamole for an extra kick.
5. **Enjoy**: Serve immediately as a healthy snack or appetizer.

Prep Time: 10 minutes

Total Time: 10 minutes

Servings: 4

Nutrition (per serving)

- Calories: 120
- Total Fat: 8g
- Saturated Fat: 1g
- Cholesterol: 0mg
- Sodium: 150mg (varies with guacamole)
- Carbohydrates: 12g
- Fiber: 4g

- Sugar: 2g
- Protein: 2g

11.1.12 Baked Kale Chips

Ingredients

- 1 bunch of curly kale (about 10 oz)
- 1-2 tablespoons olive oil (or avocado oil)
- 1 teaspoon kosher salt (or to taste)
- ½ teaspoon garlic powder (optional)
- ½ teaspoon paprika (optional)
- 2-3 tablespoons grated Parmesan cheese (optional)

Directions

1. **Preheat the Oven**: Preheat your oven to 350°F (175°C). Line a large baking sheet with parchment paper for easy cleanup.
2. **Prepare the Kale**: Wash the kale thoroughly and dry it completely using a salad spinner or by patting it with paper towels. Remove the thick stems and tear the leaves into bite-sized pieces.
3. **Season the Kale**: In a large mixing bowl, drizzle the kale pieces with olive oil and sprinkle with salt, garlic powder, and paprika if using. Toss the kale with your hands or a spoon to ensure all pieces are evenly coated.
4. **Arrange on Baking Sheet**: Spread the seasoned kale in a single layer on the prepared baking sheet. Avoid overcrowding the pan to ensure even crisping.
5. **Bake**: Bake in the preheated oven for 10-12 minutes, or until the edges are crispy and the kale is slightly browned. Keep an eye on them, as they can burn quickly.
6. **Add Cheese (Optional)**: If using Parmesan cheese, sprinkle it over the kale chips and return to the oven for an additional 3-5 minutes, until the cheese is melted and the chips are crispy.
7. **Cool and Serve**: Remove the kale chips from the oven and let them cool for about 10 minutes. They will continue to crisp up as they cool. Enjoy immediately or store in an airtight container at room temperature for up to 3 days.

Prep Time: 10 minutes

Cook Time: 15 minutes

Total Time: 25 minutes

Servings: 4

Nutrition (per serving)

- Calories: 80
- Total Fat: 7g
- Saturated Fat: 1g
- Cholesterol: 2mg (if using cheese)
- Sodium: 296mg
- Carbohydrates: 4g
- Fiber: 1g
- Sugar: 1g
- Protein: 1g

11.1.13 Cherry Tomatoes with Mozzarella

Ingredients

- 2 cups cherry tomatoes, halved
- 1 cup mozzarella balls (bocconcini or ciliegine)
- 2 tablespoons fresh basil, chopped
- 2 tablespoons olive oil
- 1 tablespoon balsamic vinegar (optional)
- Salt and pepper to taste

Directions

1. **Prepare the Ingredients**: Wash the cherry tomatoes and basil. Halve the cherry tomatoes and set them aside.
2. **Combine in a Bowl**: In a large mixing bowl, combine the halved cherry tomatoes, mozzarella balls, and chopped basil.
3. **Dress the Salad**: Drizzle the olive oil and balsamic vinegar (if using) over the mixture. Season with salt and pepper to taste.
4. **Toss Gently**: Carefully toss the ingredients together to ensure everything is well coated without breaking the mozzarella balls.
5. **Serve**: Serve immediately as a fresh salad or appetizer. You can also refrigerate it for about 30 minutes to allow the flavors to meld.

Prep Time: 10 minutes

Total Time: 10 minutes

Servings: 4

Nutrition (per serving)

- Calories: 150
- Total Fat: 10g
- Saturated Fat: 3g
- Cholesterol: 15mg

- Sodium: 200mg
- Carbohydrates: 8g
- Fiber: 1g
- Sugar: 3g
- Protein: 8g

11.1.14 Smoothie Popsicles

Ingredients

- 2 cups fresh or frozen fruit (such as strawberries, bananas, blueberries, or mango)
- 1 cup Greek yogurt or any yogurt of your choice
- 1/2 cup fruit juice (such as orange juice or apple juice) or coconut water
- 1 tablespoon honey or maple syrup (optional, depending on sweetness preference)
- 1 teaspoon vanilla extract (optional)

Directions

1. **Blend the Ingredients**: In a blender, combine the fruit, yogurt, juice, honey (if using), and vanilla extract. Blend until smooth and creamy.
2. **Taste and Adjust**: Taste the mixture and adjust the sweetness if needed by adding more honey or juice.
3. **Pour into Molds**: Pour the smoothie mixture into popsicle molds, leaving a little space at the top for expansion as they freeze.
4. **Insert Sticks**: If your molds require sticks, insert them into the mixture.
5. **Freeze**: Place the molds in the freezer and freeze for at least 4-6 hours, or until completely solid.
6. **Unmold and Serve**: To remove the popsicles, run warm water over the outside of the molds for a few seconds. Gently pull the popsicles out and enjoy!

Prep Time: 10 minutes

Total Time: 4-6 hours (freezing time)

Servings: 6-8 popsicles

Nutrition (per popsicle, based on 8 servings)

- Calories: 80
- Total Fat: 2g
- Saturated Fat: 1g

- Cholesterol: 5mg
- Sodium: 30mg
- Carbohydrates: 14g
- Fiber: 1g
- Sugar: 8g
- Protein: 3g

11.1.15 Whole Grain Crackers with Cheese

Ingredients

- 1 cup whole grain crackers (store-bought or homemade)
- 4 ounces cheese (such as cheddar, gouda, or mozzarella), sliced or cubed
- Optional toppings: fresh herbs (like basil or thyme), sliced tomatoes, or olives

Directions

1. **Prepare the Crackers**: If using homemade crackers, ensure they are baked and cooled. If using store-bought, simply have them ready on a serving plate.
2. **Slice the Cheese**: Cut the cheese into slices or cubes, depending on your preference.
3. **Assemble**: Arrange the whole grain crackers on a serving platter. Top each cracker with a slice or cube of cheese.
4. **Add Optional Toppings**: If desired, add fresh herbs, sliced tomatoes, or olives on top of the cheese for extra flavor.
5. **Serve**: Enjoy immediately as a healthy snack or appetizer.

Prep Time: 5 minutes

Total Time: 5 minutes

Servings: 4

Nutrition (per serving, based on 4 servings)

- Calories: 180
- Total Fat: 10g
- Saturated Fat: 5g
- Cholesterol: 20mg
- Sodium: 300mg
- Carbohydrates: 14g
- Fiber: 2g
- Sugar: 1g
- Protein: 8g

Desserts Recipes

11.2.1 Baked Apples with Cinnamon

Ingredients

- 4 medium-sized apples (such as Gala, Fuji, or Honeycrisp)
- 1/4 cup brown sugar
- 1 teaspoon ground cinnamon
- 1/4 teaspoon ground nutmeg (optional)
- 2 tablespoons unsalted butter, softened
- 1/4 cup chopped walnuts or pecans (optional)
- 1/4 cup raisins or dried cranberries (optional)
- Vanilla ice cream or whipped cream for serving (optional)

Directions

1. **Preheat the Oven**: Preheat your oven to 375°F (190°C).
2. **Prepare the Apples**: Wash the apples and use a sharp knife or an apple corer to remove the cores, leaving a small hole at the top. Be careful not to cut all the way through. Use a spoon to scoop out any seeds or membranes.
3. **Make the Filling**: In a small bowl, mix together the brown sugar, cinnamon, and nutmeg (if using). Spoon the mixture into the hollowed-out centers of the apples. Top each apple with a teaspoon of softened butter.
4. **Bake**: Place the stuffed apples in a baking dish and pour a small amount of water into the bottom of the dish to prevent the apples from burning. Bake for 30-40 minutes, or until the apples are tender when pierced with a fork.
5. **Add Optional Toppings**: During the last 10 minutes of baking, sprinkle the chopped nuts and raisins or cranberries over the apples, if using.

6. **Serve**: Remove the baked apples from the oven and let them cool for a few minutes. Serve warm, with a scoop of vanilla ice cream or a dollop of whipped cream if desired.

Prep Time: 10 minutes

Cook Time: 40 minutes

Total Time: 50 minutes

Servings: 4

Nutrition (per serving)

- Calories: 200
- Total Fat: 7g
- Saturated Fat: 3g
- Cholesterol: 10mg
- Sodium: 0mg
- Carbohydrates: 35g
- Fiber: 5g
- Sugar: 28g
- Protein: 1g

11.2.2 Lemon Sorbet

Ingredients

- 1 cup freshly squeezed lemon juice (about 6-8 lemons)
- 1 cup water
- 3/4 cup granulated sugar
- 1 tablespoon grated lemon zest (optional)

Directions

1. **In a medium saucepan**, combine the water and sugar. Heat over medium, stirring occasionally, until the sugar has completely dissolved. Remove from heat and let cool to room temperature.
2. **In a large bowl**, whisk together the cooled sugar syrup, lemon juice, and lemon zest (if using).
3. **Pour the mixture into a shallow metal baking pan** and place in the freezer. Freeze for 1 hour, then remove and stir vigorously with a fork to break up any ice crystals that have formed around the edges.
4. **Return to the freezer and freeze for another hour**. Repeat this process of stirring and breaking up the ice crystals every hour until the sorbet is frozen and creamy, about 3-4 hours total.
5. **Once fully frozen, scoop the sorbet into individual serving dishes or glasses.** Garnish with lemon slices or mint leaves if desired.
6. **Serve immediately** or store in an airtight container in the freezer for up to 2 weeks.

Prep Time: 10 minutes

Cook Time: 5 minutes

Total Time: 3-4 hours (including freezing time)

Servings: 4-6

Nutrition (per serving, based on 6 servings)

- Calories: 120
- Total Fat: 0g
- Saturated Fat: 0g
- Cholesterol: 0mg
- Sodium: 0mg
- Carbohydrates: 31g
- Fiber: 0g
- Sugar: 29g
- Protein: 0g

11.2.3 Berry Compote with Angel Food Cake

Ingredients

For the Berry Compote:

- 2 cups mixed berries (such as strawberries, blueberries, and raspberries)
- 1/4 cup granulated sugar (adjust based on berry sweetness)
- 1 tablespoon lemon juice
- 1 teaspoon vanilla extract (optional)

For the Angel Food Cake:

- 1 store-bought angel food cake or homemade (about 10 inches)
- Whipped cream for serving (optional)
- Fresh mint leaves for garnish (optional)

Directions

1. **Prepare the Berry Compote**:
    - In a medium saucepan, combine the mixed berries, sugar, lemon juice, and vanilla extract (if using).
    - Cook over medium heat, stirring gently until the berries start to release their juices and the mixture begins to simmer, about 5-10 minutes.
    - Remove from heat and let the compote cool slightly. It will thicken as it cools.
2. **Prepare the Angel Food Cake**:
    - If using a store-bought cake, slice it into individual servings. If making from scratch, allow it to cool completely before slicing.
3. **Assemble the Dessert**:
    - Place a slice of angel food cake on a serving plate.
    - Spoon the warm berry compote generously over the cake.
    - Top with a dollop of whipped cream if desired.

4. **Garnish**:
    - Add fresh mint leaves for a pop of color and extra flavor.
5. **Serve**: Enjoy immediately while the compote is warm.

Prep Time: 10 minutes

Cook Time: 10 minutes

Total Time: 20 minutes

Servings: 8

Nutrition (per serving, based on 8 servings)

- Calories: 150
- Total Fat: 1g
- Saturated Fat: 0g
- Cholesterol: 0mg
- Sodium: 50mg
- Carbohydrates: 34g
- Fiber: 2g
- Sugar: 20g
- Protein: 3g

11.2.4 Low-Sugar Rice Pudding

Ingredients

- **1 cup** instant rice
- **3 cups** low-fat milk
- **1/3 cup** monk fruit sweetener with erythritol
- **1/4 teaspoon** cinnamon
- **1/2 teaspoon** vanilla extract
- **2 large** eggs

Directions

1. **Combine Ingredients:** In a saucepan, mix the low-fat milk, instant rice, monk fruit sweetener, and cinnamon. Bring the mixture to a boil over medium heat.
2. **Simmer:** Once boiling, reduce the heat and let it simmer for about **6 minutes**, stirring occasionally.
3. **Prepare Egg Mixture:** While the rice is simmering, whisk together the eggs and vanilla extract in a separate bowl.
4. **Temper the Eggs:** Gradually add a small amount of the hot rice mixture to the egg mixture while stirring continuously. Repeat this process until the egg mixture is warmed.
5. **Combine Mixtures:** Slowly pour the egg mixture back into the saucepan with the rice and milk mixture. Stir continuously until the pudding starts to thicken.
6. **Thicken Further:** Remove from heat and let the pudding sit for about **30 minutes** to thicken further.
7. **Serve:** Optionally, top with whipped cream and fresh fruit before serving.

Cooking and Prep Time

- **Prep Time:** 5 minutes
- **Cook Time:** 10 minutes
- **Total Time:** 45 minutes (including thickening time)

Serving

This recipe yields approximately **4 servings**.

Nutrition Information (per serving)

- **Calories:** 203
- **Weight Watchers Personal Points:** 5

11.2.5 Pineapple Upside-Down Cake

Ingredients

For the Topping:

- **6 tablespoons** unsalted butter, melted
- **⅔ cup** light brown sugar, packed
- **1 (20 oz.) can** pineapple rings in juice (about 11 slices), drained and patted dry
- **11** maraschino cherries

For the Cake Batter:

- **4 tablespoons** unsalted butter, softened
- **½ cup + 2 tablespoons** granulated sugar
- **2 large** eggs, at room temperature
- **½ teaspoon** vanilla extract
- **1½ cups** all-purpose flour
- **1½ teaspoons** baking powder
- **¼ teaspoon** salt
- **½ cup** heavy whipping cream
- **¼ cup** milk

Directions

1. **Preheat the Oven:** Preheat your oven to 350°F (180°C).
2. **Prepare the Topping:** In a 9-inch round cake pan, pour the melted butter and sprinkle the brown sugar evenly over the bottom. Arrange the pineapple rings on top of the sugar and place a maraschino cherry in the center of each pineapple ring. Set aside.
3. **Make the Cake Batter:** In a mixing bowl, cream together the softened butter and granulated sugar until light and fluffy. Add the eggs one at a time, mixing well after each addition. Stir in the vanilla extract.

4. **Combine Dry Ingredients:** In another bowl, whisk together the flour, baking powder, and salt. Gradually add this dry mixture to the wet mixture, alternating with the heavy cream and milk. Mix until just combined.
5. **Pour and Bake:** Pour the cake batter over the arranged pineapple and cherries in the pan. Smooth the top with a spatula. Bake in the preheated oven for about **35-40 minutes**, or until a toothpick inserted into the center comes out clean.
6. **Cool and Serve:** Allow the cake to cool in the pan for about **5 minutes** before inverting it onto a serving plate. Serve warm or at room temperature.

Cooking and Prep Time

- **Prep Time:** 15 minutes
- **Cook Time:** 35-40 minutes
- **Total Time:** Approximately 55-60 minutes

Serving

This recipe yields about **8 servings**.

Nutrition Information (per serving)

- **Calories:** Approximately 290
- **Total Fat:** 12g
- **Saturated Fat:** 7g
- **Cholesterol:** 70mg
- **Sodium:** 200mg
- **Total Carbohydrates:** 42g
- **Dietary Fiber:** 1g
- **Sugars:** 24g
- **Protein:** 3g

11.2.6 Poached Pears with Vanilla

Ingredients

- **6 cups** water
- **1 cup** granulated sugar
- **1** vanilla bean, split lengthwise
- **4** ripe but firm pears, peeled, stems left intact
- **1 teaspoon** vanilla extract

Directions

1. In a large saucepan, combine the water, sugar, and vanilla bean. Bring to a simmer over medium heat, stirring occasionally until the sugar has dissolved.
2. Add the peeled pears to the simmering liquid. If needed, place a small plate or lid on top of the pears to keep them submerged. Reduce heat to low and simmer for 20-30 minutes, turning the pears occasionally, until they are tender when pierced with a knife.
3. Using a slotted spoon, transfer the poached pears to a serving dish. Remove the vanilla bean from the poaching liquid.
4. Continue simmering the poaching liquid for 10-15 minutes until reduced by about half and slightly thickened. Remove from heat and stir in the vanilla extract.
5. Pour the warm vanilla sauce over the poached pears. Serve warm, at room temperature, or chilled. Garnish with a sprinkle of cinnamon or a dollop of whipped cream if desired.

Cooking and Prep Time

- **Prep Time:** 10 minutes
- **Cook Time:** 30-45 minutes
- **Total Time:** 40-55 minutes

Serving

This recipe yields 4 servings.

Nutrition Information (per serving)

- **Calories:** 280
- **Total Fat:** 0g
- **Saturated Fat:** 0g
- **Cholesterol:** 0mg
- **Sodium:** 10mg
- **Total Carbohydrates:** 73g
- **Dietary Fiber:** 5g
- **Sugars:** 64g
- **Protein:** 1g

11.2.7 Almond Flour Cookies

Ingredients

- **2 cups** blanched almond flour
- **2 large** eggs
- **1/2 cup** butter or coconut oil, softened
- **1/2 cup** coconut sugar
- **1 teaspoon** vanilla extract
- **1/2 teaspoon** baking soda
- **1/4 teaspoon** salt
- **1/2 cup** dark chocolate chips or chopped dark chocolate

Directions

1. Preheat your oven to 350°F (175°C). Line a baking sheet with parchment paper.
2. In a large mixing bowl, cream together the softened butter (or coconut oil) and coconut sugar until smooth and well combined. Beat in the eggs one at a time, then stir in the vanilla extract.
3. In a separate bowl, whisk together the almond flour, baking soda, and salt. Gradually add the dry ingredients to the wet ingredients and mix until just combined. Fold in the chocolate chips.
4. Scoop the dough by the tablespoon onto the prepared baking sheet, spacing them about 2 inches apart. Gently press down on each cookie to flatten slightly.
5. Bake for 9-11 minutes, or until the cookies are lightly golden around the edges. They will be very soft when warm. Allow them to cool on the baking sheet for 5 minutes before transferring to a wire rack to cool completely.

Cooking and Prep Time

- **Prep Time:** 10 minutes
- **Cook Time:** 9-11 minutes
- **Total Time:** 20-25 minutes

Serving

This recipe yields approximately 24 cookies.

Nutrition Information (per cookie)

- **Calories:** 120
- **Total Fat:** 9g
- **Saturated Fat:** 4g
- **Cholesterol:** 25mg
- **Sodium:** 70mg
- **Total Carbohydrates:** 9g
- **Dietary Fiber:** 2g
- **Sugars:** 6g
- **Protein:** 3g

11.2.8 Mango Sorbet

Ingredients

- **3 ripe mangoes**, peeled and pitted
- **1/2 cup** granulated sugar (adjust based on sweetness preference)
- **1/4 cup** fresh lime juice
- **1/2 cup** water (optional, for blending)
- **Pinch of salt** (optional)

Directions

1. **Prepare the Mangoes:** Cut the mangoes into chunks and place them in a blender or food processor.
2. **Blend Ingredients:** Add the sugar, lime juice, and a splash of water (if needed) to help with blending. Blend until the mixture is smooth and creamy.
3. **Taste and Adjust:** Taste the mixture and adjust sweetness by adding more sugar or lime juice if desired.
4. **Freeze the Mixture:** Pour the mango mixture into a shallow dish or a loaf pan. Cover and freeze for about **4-6 hours**, or until solid.
5. **Serve:** Before serving, let the sorbet sit at room temperature for about 5-10 minutes to soften slightly. Scoop into bowls and enjoy!

Prep Time

- **Prep Time:** 10 minutes
- **Freeze Time:** 4-6 hours (or until solid)

Serving

This recipe yields approximately **4 servings**.

Nutrition Information (per serving)

- **Calories:** 150
- **Total Fat:** 0g
- **Saturated Fat:** 0g

- **Cholesterol:** 0mg
- **Sodium:** 5mg
- **Total Carbohydrates:** 38g
- **Dietary Fiber:** 2g
- **Sugars:** 30g
- **Protein:** 1g

11.2.9 Low-Sugar Banana Bread

Ingredients

- 4 ripe bananas (about 1 ⅓ cups, mashed)
- 1 large egg
- 1 tablespoon vanilla extract
- 3 tablespoons light brown sugar
- 2 tablespoons granulated sugar
- 1 teaspoon ground cinnamon
- 1 teaspoon baking powder
- 1 teaspoon baking soda
- ½ teaspoon salt
- 1 ½ cups all-purpose flour (can substitute with whole wheat flour)
- 2 tablespoons unsalted butter, melted (or substitute with applesauce)

Directions

1. **Preheat the Oven**: Preheat your oven to 350°F (175°C). Grease a standard 9x5-inch loaf pan, optionally lining the bottom with parchment paper for easier removal.
2. **Prepare the Banana Mixture**: In a large mixing bowl, mash the bananas until smooth. Add the egg, vanilla extract, brown sugar, granulated sugar, and cinnamon. Stir well to combine.
3. **Mix Dry Ingredients**: In a separate bowl, whisk together the flour, baking powder, baking soda, and salt.
4. **Combine Mixtures**: Gradually add the dry ingredients to the banana mixture, stirring until just combined. Gently fold in the melted butter.
5. **Bake**: Pour the batter into the prepared loaf pan. Bake for 35-45 minutes, or until a toothpick inserted into the center comes out clean.
6. **Cool**: Allow the bread to cool in the pan for 5-10 minutes before transferring it to a wire rack to cool completely.

Cooking and Prep Time

- **Prep Time**: 10 minutes
- **Cook Time**: 35-45 minutes
- **Total Time**: Approximately 1 hour

Serving

This recipe yields about 8-10 slices, making it perfect for sharing or enjoying throughout the week.

Nutritional Information (per slice, approximately)

- **Calories**: 100
- **Total Fat**: 3g
- **Saturated Fat**: 1g
- **Cholesterol**: 20mg
- **Sodium**: 150mg
- **Total Carbohydrates**: 20g
- **Dietary Fiber**: 1g
- **Sugars**: 6g
- **Protein**: 2g

11.2.10 Chia Seed Pudding

Ingredients

For a basic chia seed pudding (serves 4):

- ½ cup chia seeds
- 2 cups unsweetened plant-based milk (such as almond, coconut, or soy)
- 1-2 tablespoons maple syrup (adjust to taste)
- ½ teaspoon vanilla extract (optional)
- ½ teaspoon cinnamon (optional)

Optional Toppings:

- Fresh fruits (berries, bananas, mango)
- Nuts and seeds
- Granola
- Coconut flakes
- Additional maple syrup or honey

Directions

1. **Combine Ingredients**: In a large bowl or jar, mix the chia seeds, milk, maple syrup, vanilla extract, and cinnamon. Stir well to ensure the chia seeds are evenly distributed.
2. **Initial Rest**: Let the mixture sit for about 10 minutes. This allows the chia seeds to start absorbing the liquid and begin to gel.
3. **Stir Again**: After 10 minutes, stir the mixture again to break up any clumps of chia seeds.
4. **Chill**: Cover the bowl or jar and refrigerate for at least 1 hour, or overnight for a thicker consistency.
5. **Serve**: Once the pudding has thickened, stir it again before serving. Top with your favorite fruits, nuts, or other toppings.

Cooking and Prep Time

- **Prep Time**: 10 minutes
- **Chill Time**: 1 hour (or overnight)
- **Total Time**: Approximately 1 hour and 10 minutes (or overnight)

Serving

This recipe yields about 4 servings, making it perfect for meal prep or sharing.

Nutritional Information (per serving, approximately)

- **Calories**: 150
- **Total Fat**: 7g
- **Saturated Fat**: 1g
- **Cholesterol**: 0mg
- **Sodium**: 50mg
- **Total Carbohydrates**: 16g
- **Dietary Fiber**: 10g
- **Sugars**: 4g
- **Protein**: 5g

11.2.11 Strawberry Shortcake

Ingredients

For the Strawberries:

- 6–7 cups fresh strawberries, quartered
- 1/4 cup + 2 tablespoons (75g) granulated sugar, divided
- 1 teaspoon pure vanilla extract

For the Biscuits:

- 2 3/4 cups (345g) all-purpose flour, plus extra for dusting
- 1/4 cup (50g) granulated sugar
- 4 teaspoons baking powder
- 1/2 teaspoon baking soda
- 1 teaspoon salt
- 3/4 cup (12 tablespoons; 170g) cold unsalted butter, cubed
- 1 cup (240ml) cold buttermilk

For the Whipped Cream:

- 1 cup (240ml) heavy cream
- 2 tablespoons granulated sugar
- 1 teaspoon vanilla extract

Directions

1. **Prepare the Strawberries**: In a large bowl, combine the quartered strawberries with 1/4 cup of sugar and vanilla extract. Mix well and let sit for about 30 minutes to macerate, allowing the strawberries to release their juices.
2. **Make the Biscuits**:
    - Preheat your oven to 425°F (220°C).
    - In a large bowl, whisk together the flour, 1/4 cup sugar, baking powder, baking soda, and salt.

- Cut in the cold butter using a pastry cutter or your fingers until the mixture resembles coarse crumbs.
- Stir in the cold buttermilk until just combined. Do not overmix.
- Turn the dough onto a floured surface and gently knead it a few times. Pat it into a rectangle about 1-inch thick.
- Cut into rounds using a biscuit cutter and place on a baking sheet lined with parchment paper.

3. **Bake the Biscuits**: Bake in the preheated oven for 12-15 minutes or until golden brown. Remove from the oven and let cool slightly.
4. **Prepare the Whipped Cream**: In a medium bowl, beat the heavy cream, sugar, and vanilla extract with an electric mixer until soft peaks form.
5. **Assemble the Shortcakes**: Slice the biscuits in half horizontally. Spoon a generous amount of macerated strawberries over the bottom half, add a dollop of whipped cream, and place the top half of the biscuit on top. Serve immediately.

Cooking and Prep Time

- **Prep Time**: 20 minutes
- **Cook Time**: 15 minutes
- **Total Time**: Approximately 35 minutes (plus 30 minutes for strawberries to macerate)

Serving

This recipe makes about 8 servings, depending on the size of the biscuits.

Nutritional Information (per serving, approximately)

- **Calories**: 320
- **Total Fat**: 18g
- **Saturated Fat**: 10g
- **Cholesterol**: 60mg
- **Sodium**: 250mg
- **Total Carbohydrates**: 36g

- **Dietary Fiber**: 2g
- **Sugars**: 10g
- **Protein**: 4g

11.2.12 Apricot Bars

Ingredients

For the Filling:

- 2 lbs (910g) fresh apricots, pitted and halved (or 30 oz canned apricots, drained)
- 3/4 cup (150g) granulated sugar (adjust to taste)
- 1 tablespoon (15ml) orange liqueur (optional, such as Grand Marnier)

For the Crust and Topping:

- 1 cup (125g) all-purpose flour
- 1/2 cup (110g) packed brown sugar
- 1/4 teaspoon kosher salt
- 1/4 teaspoon baking soda
- 1/2 cup (113g) cold unsalted butter, cut into small cubes
- 1 cup (90g) old-fashioned oats

Directions

1. **Prepare the Apricot Filling**: In a medium saucepan, combine the apricots and granulated sugar. Cook over medium heat until the sugar dissolves and the apricots soften (about 5-10 minutes). If using fresh apricots, you may need to cook longer. Stir in the orange liqueur if using. Remove from heat and let cool slightly.
2. **Make the Apricot Puree**: Transfer the cooked apricots to a blender or food processor and puree until smooth. Set aside to cool completely.
3. **Preheat the Oven**: Preheat your oven to 350°F (175°C). Grease a 9x13-inch baking dish or line it with parchment paper.
4. **Prepare the Crust and Topping**: In a large bowl, whisk together the flour, brown sugar, salt, and baking soda. Cut in the cold butter until the mixture resembles coarse crumbs. Stir in the oats until evenly combined.

5. **Assemble the Bars**: Press about two-thirds of the crust mixture into the bottom of the prepared baking dish to form an even layer. Spread the apricot puree over the crust, then sprinkle the remaining crust mixture on top.
6. **Bake**: Bake in the preheated oven for 50-65 minutes, or until the top is golden brown.
7. **Cool and Serve**: Allow the bars to cool in the pan before slicing into squares. Store any leftovers in the refrigerator.

Cooking and Prep Time

- **Prep Time**: 20 minutes
- **Cook Time**: 50-65 minutes
- **Total Time**: Approximately 1 hour and 15 minutes

Serving

This recipe yields about 12-16 bars, making it great for sharing at gatherings or enjoying as a snack.

Nutritional Information (per bar, approximately)

- **Calories**: 180
- **Total Fat**: 8g
- **Saturated Fat**: 4g
- **Cholesterol**: 20mg
- **Sodium**: 50mg
- **Total Carbohydrates**: 27g
- **Dietary Fiber**: 2g
- **Sugars**: 10g
- **Protein**: 3g

11.2.13 Coconut Macaroons

Ingredients

- 1 (14-oz.) bag sweetened flaked coconut (about 5 ⅓ cups)
- 1 (14-oz.) can sweetened condensed milk
- 1 tablespoon vanilla extract
- 2 large egg whites (optional for a lighter texture)
- 1/4 teaspoon salt (if using egg whites)
- 4 ounces semi-sweet chocolate (optional for dipping)

Directions

1. **Preheat the Oven**: Preheat your oven to 350°F (175°C). Line a baking sheet with parchment paper or a Silpat mat.
2. **Combine Ingredients**: In a large bowl, mix together the sweetened flaked coconut, sweetened condensed milk, and vanilla extract until well combined. If using egg whites, beat them separately until stiff peaks form and then fold them into the coconut mixture.
3. **Form the Macaroons**: Using a small ice cream scoop or two spoons, scoop out about 1 ½ tablespoons of the mixture and place them onto the prepared baking sheet, spacing them about 2 inches apart.
4. **Bake**: Bake in the preheated oven for 15-18 minutes, or until the macaroons are golden brown.
5. **Cool**: Remove the macaroons from the oven and let them cool on the baking sheet for about 5 minutes before transferring them to a wire rack to cool completely.
6. **Optional Chocolate Dip**: If desired, melt the chocolate in a microwave-safe bowl or over a double boiler. Dip the bottoms of the cooled macaroons in the melted chocolate and return them to the baking sheet to set. You can also drizzle chocolate over the tops for decoration.

Cooking and Prep Time

- **Prep Time**: 10 minutes
- **Cook Time**: 15-18 minutes
- **Total Time**: Approximately 25-30 minutes

Serving

This recipe yields about 12-16 macaroons, depending on the size.

Nutritional Information (per macaroon, approximately)

- **Calories**: 78
- **Total Fat**: 3g
- **Saturated Fat**: 3g
- **Cholesterol**: 3mg
- **Sodium**: 40mg
- **Total Carbohydrates**: 10g
- **Dietary Fiber**: 1g
- **Sugars**: 9g
- **Protein**: 1g

11.2.14 Chocolate Avocado Mousse

Ingredients

- 2 medium ripe avocados (pitted and peeled)
- 6–7 tablespoons unsweetened cocoa powder
- 6–8 tablespoons pure maple syrup (adjust to taste)
- 6–8 tablespoons unsweetened almond milk (or your favorite plant-based milk)
- 1 ½–2 teaspoons vanilla extract
- 1/8–1/4 teaspoon salt

Directions

1. **Blend the Ingredients**: In a food processor or high-speed blender, add the avocado flesh, cocoa powder, maple syrup, almond milk, vanilla extract, and salt.
2. **Process Until Smooth**: Blend the mixture until it is completely smooth and creamy. You may need to stop and scrape down the sides to ensure everything is well combined. Taste the mousse and adjust sweetness by adding more maple syrup if desired.
3. **Chill**: Transfer the mousse to an airtight container and refrigerate for at least 1 hour to allow the flavors to meld and the mousse to thicken.
4. **Serve**: Once chilled, spoon the mousse into serving dishes. You can garnish with fresh berries, coconut whipped cream, or chocolate shavings if desired.

Cooking and Prep Time

- **Prep Time**: 10 minutes
- **Chill Time**: 1 hour (minimum)
- **Total Time**: Approximately 1 hour and 10 minutes

Serving

This recipe yields about 4 servings, depending on portion size.

Nutritional Information (per serving, approximately)

- **Calories**: 180

- **Total Fat**: 9g
- **Saturated Fat**: 1.5g
- **Cholesterol**: 0mg
- **Sodium**: 50mg
- **Total Carbohydrates**: 23g
- **Dietary Fiber**: 6g
- **Sugars**: 10g
- **Protein**: 2g

11.2.15 Berry Tart

Ingredients

For the Crust:

- 1 ¼ cups (175g) all-purpose flour
- ½ teaspoon salt
- 1 tablespoon (15g) granulated sugar
- ½ cup (113g) unsalted butter, chilled and cut into small cubes
- 3-4 tablespoons ice water

For the Filling:

- 1 ½ pounds mixed fresh berries (such as strawberries, blueberries, raspberries, or blackberries)
- ¼ cup (50g) granulated sugar (adjust based on berry sweetness)
- 1 tablespoon cornstarch
- 1 tablespoon lemon juice
- 1 teaspoon vanilla extract (optional)

Directions

1. **Prepare the Crust**:
    - In a mixing bowl, combine the flour, salt, and sugar. Add the chilled butter and mix until the mixture resembles coarse crumbs.
    - Gradually add ice water, one tablespoon at a time, mixing until the dough just comes together. Avoid overmixing.
    - Shape the dough into a disk, wrap it in plastic wrap, and refrigerate for at least 30 minutes.
2. **Preheat the Oven**: Preheat your oven to 350°F (175°C).
3. **Roll Out the Dough**: On a floured surface, roll out the chilled dough to fit a 9-inch tart pan. Press the dough into the pan and trim any excess. Prick the bottom with a fork to prevent bubbling.

4. **Blind Bake the Crust**: Line the crust with parchment paper and fill it with pie weights or dried beans. Bake for 15 minutes, then remove the weights and parchment. Bake for an additional 10-15 minutes or until golden brown. Let it cool completely.
5. **Prepare the Filling**:
    - In a large bowl, combine the mixed berries, sugar, cornstarch, lemon juice, and vanilla extract. Gently toss to coat the berries.
6. **Assemble the Tart**: Once the crust has cooled, pour the berry mixture into the crust, spreading it evenly.
7. **Bake the Tart**: Bake the tart in the preheated oven for about 30-35 minutes, or until the filling is bubbly and the berries are tender.
8. **Cool and Serve**: Allow the tart to cool on a wire rack. Serve at room temperature or chilled, optionally with whipped cream or ice cream.

Cooking and Prep Time

- **Prep Time**: 30 minutes (plus chilling time)
- **Cook Time**: 45-50 minutes
- **Total Time**: Approximately 1 hour and 20 minutes (plus chilling)

Serving

This recipe yields about 8 servings, making it perfect for gatherings or family desserts.

Nutritional Information (per serving, approximately)

- **Calories**: 210
- **Total Fat**: 10g
- **Saturated Fat**: 6g
- **Cholesterol**: 30mg
- **Sodium**: 90mg
- **Total Carbohydrates**: 30g
- **Dietary Fiber**: 3g
- **Sugars**: 10g
- **Protein**: 2g

Exercise and Lifestyle Tips

12.1 Importance of Physical Activity

Physical activity plays a vital role in managing Stage 3 kidney disease and promoting overall health. Here are some key benefits:

1. Enhances Cardiovascular Health: Regular exercise helps maintain a healthy heart and blood vessels, reducing the risk of cardiovascular diseases, which are common among individuals with kidney disease.

2. Helps Control Blood Pressure: Physical activity can help lower and control blood pressure, reducing strain on the kidneys and slowing the progression of kidney disease.

3. Manages Weight: Maintaining a healthy weight through exercise can reduce the risk of diabetes and hypertension, both of which can further damage the kidneys.

4. Improves Muscle Strength and Function: Regular exercise helps maintain muscle strength, flexibility, and endurance, enhancing overall physical function and quality of life.

5. Boosts Mental Health: Exercise releases endorphins, which can improve mood and reduce stress, anxiety, and depression, all of which are common in individuals managing chronic conditions.

6. Enhances Energy Levels: Regular physical activity can increase energy levels and reduce fatigue, making daily activities easier and more enjoyable.

7. Supports Better Sleep: Engaging in regular exercise can improve sleep quality and duration, which is essential for overall health and well-being.

Guidelines for Safe Physical Activity:

- **Consult Your Doctor:** Before starting any exercise program, consult with your healthcare provider to ensure the activities are safe for your condition.
- **Start Slowly:** Begin with low-impact activities like walking, swimming, or gentle yoga, gradually increasing intensity as tolerated.
- **Stay Consistent:** Aim for at least 150 minutes of moderate-intensity exercise per week, divided into manageable sessions.
- **Listen to Your Body:** Focus on your body's signs and keep away from overexertion. Rest when needed and adjust activities based on your energy levels and any symptoms you may experience.
- **Hydrate Properly:** Ensure adequate hydration before, during, and after exercise, as advised by your healthcare provider.

Incorporating regular physical activity into your routine can significantly enhance your ability to manage Stage 3 kidney disease and improve your overall health and quality of life.

12.2 Safe Exercises for Seniors with Kidney Disease

For seniors with Stage 3 kidney disease, engaging in regular, safe physical activity is crucial for maintaining health and well-being. Here are some recommended exercises:

1. Walking:

- **Benefits:** Improves cardiovascular health, strengthens muscles, and enhances mood.
- **Tips:** Start with short distances and gradually increase duration. Use supportive footwear and choose flat, even surfaces.

2. Swimming and Water Aerobics:

- **Benefits:** Low-impact, reduces stress on joints, and provides resistance for muscle strengthening.
- **Tips:** Ensure the pool is easily accessible. Consider joining a water aerobics class tailored for seniors.

3. Chair Exercises:

- **Benefits:** Improves flexibility, strength, and circulation without the need for standing.
- **Tips:** Perform exercises like seated leg lifts, arm raises, and gentle stretches. Use a sturdy chair for support.

4. Stretching:

- **Benefits:** Enhances flexibility, reduces muscle tension, and improves range of motion.
- **Tips:** Incorporate gentle stretching into your daily routine. Hold extends for 15-30 seconds without bobbing.

5. Yoga and Tai Chi:

- **Benefits:** Promotes balance, flexibility, and relaxation. Reduces stress and enhances mental well-being.
- **Tips:** Choose beginner classes or routines specifically designed for seniors. Center around delicate developments and appropriate relaxing.

6. Strength Training:

- **Benefits:** Increases muscle strength, supports bone health, and improves functional abilities.
- **Tips:** Use light weights or resistance bands. Perform exercises like bicep curls, leg lifts, and wall push-ups. Aim for 2-3 sessions per week with rest days in between.

7. Cycling:

- **Benefits:** Enhances cardiovascular health and leg strength.
- **Tips:** Use a stationary bike for stability. Adjust the seat and resistance levels for comfort and safety.

8. Balance Exercises:

- **Benefits:** Improves stability and reduces the risk of falls.
- **Tips:** Practice standing on one foot, heel-to-toe walks, and side leg raises. Use a chair or wall for support if needed.

Incorporating these safe exercises into your routine can help manage kidney disease, improve physical fitness, and enhance overall quality of life for seniors.

Conclusion

13.1 Encouragement and Support

Managing Stage 3 kidney disease can be challenging, but with the right encouragement and support, seniors can maintain a positive outlook and better handle their condition.

1. Emotional Support: Stay connected with family, friends, and support groups. Sharing experiences and feelings can reduce stress and foster a sense of community.

2. Professional Guidance: Regularly consult with healthcare providers, including nephrologists and dietitians, to receive personalized care and advice.

3. Stay Informed: Educate yourself about kidney disease and its management. Information enables you to settle on informed conclusions about your wellbeing.

4. Healthy Lifestyle: Follow a kidney-friendly diet, engage in safe physical activities, and adhere to prescribed treatments to maintain optimal health.

5. Positive Mindset: Focus on the aspects of life that you can control and celebrate small victories. An uplifting outlook can essentially influence your prosperity.

With the right encouragement and support, seniors can navigate the challenges of Stage 3 kidney disease more effectively and maintain a fulfilling life.

13.3 Final Thoughts

Managing Stage 3 kidney disease can be a daunting journey, but with the right knowledge, support, and lifestyle changes, it is possible to live a fulfilling and healthy life. This book has provided you with essential information on understanding kidney disease, the importance of a tailored diet, and practical tips for meal planning, grocery shopping, and physical activity.

Remember, each individual's journey is unique, and it's important to work closely with your healthcare team to develop a personalized plan that meets your specific needs. Embrace the support of family, friends, and community resources, and don't hesitate to seek help when needed.

By making informed dietary choices, staying active, and maintaining a positive mindset, you can take control of your health and well-being. Little, steady changes can prompt critical enhancements in your personal satisfaction. Stay committed to your health, celebrate your progress, and remember that you have the power to make a difference in your own life.

Your journey with kidney disease is a testament to your strength and resilience. Continue to educate yourself, advocate for your health, and cherish the support around you. Here's to a healthier, happier future.